Stephen Tang is a herbalist and acupuncturist living and working in Manchester's Chinatown. Trained in Hong Kong, he and his wife carry on a long family tradition of practising Chinese herbal medicine. Martin Palmer, Director of the International Consultancy on Religion, Education and Culture, is a student of Chinese belief and proficient in Chinese.

Both live in Manchester.

RIDER

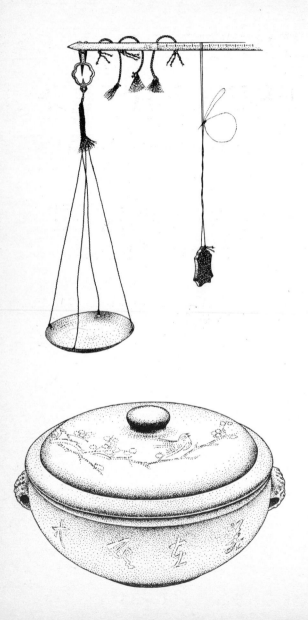

CHINESE HERBAL
PRESCRIPTIONS

A practical and authoritative

self-help guide

Stephen Tang and
Martin Palmer

RIDER
London Melbourne Auckland Johannesburg

Copyright © International Consultancy on Religion,
Education and Culture, 1986

All rights reserved

First published in 1986 by Rider & Company,
an imprint of Century Hutchinson Ltd,
Brookmount House, 62–65 Chandos Place, Covent Garden,
London WC2N 4NW

Century Hutchinson Publishing Group (Australia) Pty Ltd
16–22 Church Street, Hawthorn, Melbourne, Victoria 3122

Century Hutchinson Group (NZ) Ltd
32–34 View Road, PO Box 40–086, Glenfield, Auckland 10

Century Hutchinson Group (SA) Pty Ltd
PO Box 337, Bergvlei 2012, South Africa

Set in Plantin by Tradespools Ltd, Frome, Somerset

Printed and bound in Great Britain by
The Guernsey Press Co Ltd,
Guernsey, Channel Islands

British Library Cataloguing in Publication Data

Tang, Stephen
Chinese herbal prescriptions.
1. Materia medica, vegetable—China
2. Herbs—Therapeutic use 3. Medicine, Chinese
I. Title   II. Palmer, Martin
615'.321   RS164

ISBN 0-7126-9470-6

CONTENTS

CAUTION

While Chinese herbal medicine, in the hands of
the experienced practitioner, is often used to
treat serious and even life-threatening disease, it
should *never* be used in this way by the amateur.
Self-diagnosis and treatment should only be used
for minor ailments, and a doctor should be
consulted if a condition is persistent or if there is
abnormally high or low temperature, delirium or
any other indication that the illness is anything
more than a minor complaint.

Many of the plants used are wild ones native to
China; using other species of the same genus will
not produce the same results and may even be
dangerous.

PREFACE

Early on in the work on this book the wordprocessor, during one of the many printouts of the manuscript, made an interesting mistake. Instead of printing out 'Chinese Angelica', it printed out 'Chinese Angela'. This was a very perceptive comment by our machine, for without the assistance of Angela Smith this book would never have seen the light of day. Angela has acted as interrogator, researcher, scribe and travelling link between us. We wish to record our deep appreciation of the time, trouble and care which she has given to this book. She is now aware of parts of the body which she never even knew existed!

We also wish to express our thanks to the Chinese section team of the International Consultancy on Religion, Education and Culture (ICOREC), in particular Kwok Man Ho, Joanne O'Brien, Mr Leung and Barbara Cousins.

To the many Chinese and Western colleagues who gave advice and time over endless cups of tea and dim sum, thank you.

Finally to our families, both personal and the 'family' of Rider itself, our grateful thanks for patience and care during these last few months.

There is an ancient Chinese practice whereby you pay the doctor while you are well and stop paying him when you are ill. We hope that if this book brings you better health, you will buy more copies and pass them to friends – and thus in a new way the old practice will continue!

Stephen Tang and Martin Palmer
16 August 1985

INTRODUCTION

The materials found within this book are drawn from the personal experience and work of Stephen Tang, a practising herbalist in the city of Manchester. For many generations the Tangs have been involved with herbal medicine and it is from his family lore as well as from standard texts on herbal medicine that Stephen has drawn the material to be found within.

One major criticism of many books on Chinese herbal medicine is that they do not fully explain the cultural and psychological framework within which the practice of such medicine has arisen. This has often led to frustration on the part of Western users who have sought to apply remedies without understanding the concepts underlying the prescriptions and their preparation. Further, the question of an appropriate lifestyle has often been glossed over and this has similarly led to disappointment.

In this book we have sought to explain the milieu both spiritual and physical within which traditional Chinese herbal medicine is set. We hope that through this some appreciation of the indivisible nature of both spiritual and physical wellbeing will be found by readers.

We cannot stress strongly enough the necessity for the reader to pay attention to the warnings given in this book. The herbs and prescriptions are often in themselves not dangerous, but certain combinations have great potency and thus need to be handled with care. Chinese herbal medicine is not the cure-all of the world's physical ills. It is but one branch within the school of medicine in China and thus needs to be seen alongside other forms of treatment – especially acupuncture. If you are seriously ill, then herbal medicine will probably be irrelevant to you and you should consult a doctor. If a symptom persists, then consult a doctor. Do not use this book as an answer to all illnesses, for it is not designed to be used in this way, nor is it capable of such use.

We hope that you will enjoy better health as a result of this book and that perhaps it will help to unfold a little more of the rich and fascinating culture of China to those who would explore with an open mind.

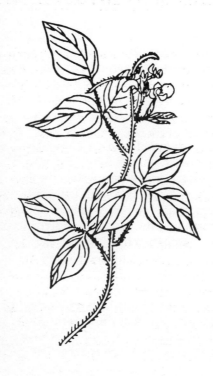

1

THE HISTORY OF CHINESE
HERBAL MEDICINE

Quite when people began consciously using herbs for medical
purposes will never be known. At some very early stage in
human history the beneficial effects of eating certain plants
must have been noticed and gradually a corpus of oral tradition
grew up around it. It seems likely, based upon archaeological
research and study of contemporary examples, that the healing
use of plants was directly linked to the key religious person in a
group. The ability to cure illness must in itself have seemed a
supernatural power, and indeed to some extent it still does,
even to sophisticated people of today. The close links between
certain diets, prescriptions and healing can still be found in
present shamanists.[1]

Shamanism is possibly the earliest world religion. The term
is used to describe the practice by which a person – the shaman
– acts as an intermediary between humans and the supernatural world. Communication takes place through ecstatic trances
and the shaman is the leading figure in the society which he
serves. The dates given for the spread of shamanism vary
enormously, but certainly go back over 8000 years. Shamanistic practices are found in Siberia (its original homeland, where,
until recently, it was commonly practised amongst the Tunga
people); in China, where it formed the basis for much of
Taoism and the early foundations of civilization; in Alaska
amongst the Inuit; and in North and South America generally,
where it has been and still is practised by the native American
population. It is obvious from this that shamanistic practices
were able to travel overland to the American continent from
Siberia during the period when these two landmasses were
linked by a bridge of ice and islands. This gives a rough latest
date of *c.* 6000 BCE, but its dissemination could have taken
place much earlier.

Whatever the age, the link between supernatural powers and herbal medicine has remained in much of Chinese life. Until this century it was simply one of the assumed principles upon which herbal medicine was based. For many overseas Chinese this link is still there.

Evidence of this shamanistic background can be found in the considerable mythology which surrounds the supposed history of herbal medicine. As with all aspects of civilization such as marriage, agriculture, divination and writing, the legends point back first to Fu-hsi, the first of the Three August Ones. These semi-divine, semi-human figures reputedly descended to Earth from Heaven to teach primitive humans how to live. Of these, the greatest is Fu-hsi, who is reputed to have lived over 4000 years ago. Shen-nung, the last of the Three August Ones, is also credited with inventing medicine, but of particular interest to us is that he is specifically described as inventing herbal medicine. He is also strongly linked with agriculture and was in fact the main deity worshipped by the emperors at the start of the agricultural year until early this century. Perhaps this link with agriculture gives a hint as to why he is also associated with the creation of specifically herb-based medicine.

Now, although Fu-hsi and Shen-nung are of interest, it is not with them that the story really starts. (Indeed, Fu-hsi has often been credited with inventing just about everything.) It is with a third great legendary figure that the details begin to emerge and some clues are to be discerned. This figure is the Yellow Emperor – Huang-ti – first of the Five August Emperors, who is supposed to have reigned from about 2697 to 2597 BCE. To him is credited the systematic development and ordering of medicine in general, for he is seen as the author of the earliest-known classical treatise on medicine, the *Huang-ti Nei Ching Su Wen* (*The Yellow Emperor's Classic of Internal Medicine*).[2] The book actually dates from somewhere around 200–100 BCE, although parts are clearly older and may go back to the early Chou dynasty (1028–722 BCE) or even to the Shang dynasty (*c.* 1523–1028 BCE). There is some evidence that Huang-ti is based on a real person – a powerful religio-political leader who imposed certain codes of law and possibly of religion upon a small but unified area of land. If so, then the idea that, under his rule, medicine became established with its own traditions and practices is not totally absurd. Some have even seen Huang-ti as a possible shaman who, through his control of the supernatural, was able to bring some unity of purpose and social organization to groups living in the Yellow River basin in China.

Given the strong links between shamanism and herbal medicine, it is not without significance that both Shen-nung and Huang-ti (and occasionally Fu-hsi as well) are depicted wearing cloaks of leaves and holding plants in their hands. The wearing of such cloaks is often found to be a sign of shamanistic practice amongst those communities who still retain shamans.

There is really little more that can be said about these three legendary figures. They merge into the mists of history and myth and will probably constantly defy our attempts either to verify them or to dismiss them. Suffice it to say that herbal medicine was, almost beyond doubt, being practised in some form over 4000 years ago and that in these legends we hear distant, indistinct echoes of some of the practitioners. For the bulk of Chinese herbalists down the centuries the figures of Fu-hsi, Shen-nung and particularly Huang-ti have been symbols of the divine accuracy and propriety of their practice.

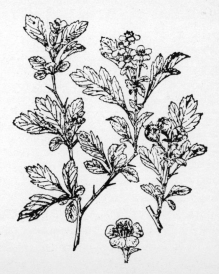

From the period of the Three August Ones and the Five August Emperors (c. 3000–2000 BCE) to the time of the earliest surviving herbal texts c. 300–200 BCE there are but brief glimpses of herbal medicine. These have to be quarried from the ancient materials contained within the Five Classics[3] and in Ssu-ma Ch'ien's *History*[4] (c. 90 BCE). One of the most revealing and human of these glimpses is found in the *Shu Ching (The Book of Historical Documents)*.[5] Compiled in its current form c. 350 BCE, much of it can be assigned to the latter half of the second millenium BCE – from 1500 to 1000. Our earliest glimpse thus comes from this time. In 1323 BCE the Emperor Wu-ting came to the throne of the Shang dynasty. In his commission to his Prime Minister Yue, Wu-ting says the following: 'Open your mind, and enrich my mind. Be you like medicine, which, if it do not distress the patient, will not cure his sickness.'[6]

How very immediate is this earliest historical statement on medicine – which for the Chinese obviously includes herbal medicine. Perhaps every culture has such a statement. We can feel confident that this is an account which is as old as the fourteenth century BCE. A thousand years later the Confucian philosopher Meng Tzu (known in the West as Mencius) quotes the *Shu Ching* thus: '*The Book of History* [the *Shu Ching*] says, "If the medicine does not make the head swim, the illness will not be cured." '[7] The same quotation also appears in the *Kuo Yu (The Discourse on the States)*.[8] This document was compiled somewhere between 770 and 476 BCE but, like the *Shu Ching*, draws on earlier documents. In this case a lost book is cited – *The Book of Wu-ting*. So many references, constantly leading back to Wu-ting, seem to provide strong evidence that this quotation actually does come down to us over 3300 years from Wu-ting himself.

Another glimpse of medicine in use or, rather, in this case not in use, comes from the year 580 BCE. It is recorded in the *Tso Chuan*, a commentary on Confucius's work *Ch'un Ch'iu (The Spring and Autumn Annals)*, which is one of the Five Classics, that the Duke of Chin became very ill and asked the duke of the neighbouring country, called, confusingly, Ch'in, to send a physician.

The Duke of Ch'in sent the physician Huan to see what he could do for him. Before he came, the Duke dreamt that there were two boys in his body. One said to the other, 'This is a clever doctor; I am afraid he will hurt us. How can we avoid him?' The other one said, 'If we take up our position above the heart and below the throat, then what can he do to us?'

When the doctor arrived he said, 'Nothing can be done to cure this illness. Its seat is above the heart and below the throat. If I try medicine, it will be of no use. If I try to pierce it [acupuncture], I will not reach it. Nothing can be done for it.'[9]

Apparently the duke was so impressed with this doctor's honesty and accuracy that he loaded him with gifts. The duke died shortly after.

There are other instances from this period on to the end of the Chou dynasty and the era of the Warring States (ends 221 BCE) which all show that the regular and regularized use of medicine by professional doctors was an accepted part of life.

Before we consider the theory and practice of herbal medicine, we should mention a parallel development. This is the mythology which found its expression in the Ministry of Medicine, part of the hierarchy of Heaven. Under the umbrella of this Taoist structure come not only the three legendary figures we have already encountered – Fu-hsi, Shen-nung and Huang-ti – but also a whole host of other deities. These deities are sometimes purely mythological – such as Yao Wang, King of Medicinal Herbs – and sometimes historical or semi-historical. For instance, there is I-yin who is reputed to have invented herbal medicinal soup around 1500 BCE. There is the famous Chou-dynasty physician Pien Ch'io, about whom there are many stories, some of which are recorded in Ssu-ma Ch'ien's *History*. The habit of deifying successful doctors continued after the fall of the Empire in 1911. According to the sinologist Henri Doré, the last such deification took place in 1913.[10] While it is difficult in some cases to date accurately or even to verify the existence of these doctor deities, there is enough evidence to show that a stream of oral tradition preserved the names of great doctors who had specialized in certain fields. Amongst these are many herbal doctors, the greatest of whom was Hua To, of whom more later.

It is in the compilation of the *Huang-ti Nei Ching Su Wen*

that we first encounter the long history of documentary evidence of the actual methods and prescriptions used in herbal medicine. This volume, first written down *c*. 200–100 BCE, has been much copied and later commentaries have become part of the core text. Nevertheless, we can still turn to it as containing some of the earliest, if not the earliest, extant details of herbal medicine. Readers will find that most of the details from the *Nei Ching* tally exactly with the methods and types of prescription included in this present book. In Book 4, Parts 13 and 14, the following is found in a discussion of methods of curing the 'five illnesses of numbness':

When this ten-day treatment did not terminate the disease, they prescribed thyme and roots of herbs. And when the stalks and roots did not show any alleviating effect, the topmost branches and the farthest roots, swallowed as medicines, were considered effective in the termination of the evil influences. [To this Wang Ping (the main commentator – *c*. 760 CE) adds that these roots and branches should be simmered or fried in oil.]

The Yellow Emperor asked, 'How can one prepare soups and clear liquids, and even lees of wine and sweet wine from the five kinds of grain?' [The five kinds are glutinous millet, wheat, millet, rice and beans.]

The great physician, Ch'i Po, answers by telling how to steam the soups, how to cut herbs at the correct time, and how in this corrupted world people must now take soups and liquid medicines.[11]

The regulating of Chinese medicine is first recorded around the time the *Nei Ching* was being compiled. In the *Ch'ien Han Shu* and the *Hou Han Shou* (*The Books of the Han*)[12] – dynastic records of the Han period (207 BCE–220 CE) – medical books were classified under four categories. First there were those books concerned with the internal structures of the body and the causes of illness. These were classed as the 'I Ching' ('I' means 'medical', not to be confused with the *I Ching – The Book of Changes*). Next there were the works on prescriptions and remedies, many of which were concerned with herbal medicine. These were called the 'Ching Fang' (meaning 'Collection of Prescriptions'). Thirdly there were the books on sexual techniques and health, known as the 'Fang Chung'. Finally there were the 'Shen Hsien' ('Ways of Gaining

Immortality') which sought relief from sickness in transcending the earthly life. In all, some thirty-six separate books are recorded under these four classifications.

By the time of the Ming dynasty (1368–1644 CE) the number of classifications had increased to thirteen. At the end of the last dynasty, the Ch'ing (1644–1911), the number of categories had been reduced to nine which were officially recognized by the Imperial Medical College.

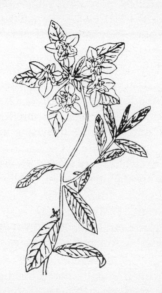

Chang Chung Ching, the great codifier of medicine who lived during the later Han times (c. 160–200 CE), laid a more systematic basis for medicine in general (developing the theory of yin and yang, for instance) and gave very detailed descriptions of symptoms and herbal remedies in his main work, the *Shang Han Lun* (*Treatise on Febrile Diseases*).[13] In this same period Hua To (c. 140–200 CE) developed hydrotherapy in general and herbal baths in particular. Hua To was probably the greatest doctor of antiquity and is honoured as such in the heavenly Ministry of Medicine. He is particularly revered by herbalists and there is still an annual herbal fair in Hubei province in his honour. Thus we can see that the Han era was a time of great systematization of herbal medicine.

However, there is a subcurrent to herbal medicine which is equally important. This was the old line of the shamans which re-emerged in the form of the main leaders and founders of religious Taoism. Many people are familiar with philososphical Taoism, known as Tao Chia (the School of Tao). At its centre lies the profound and mysterious book the *Tao Te Ching*, thought to have been written by a sage called Lao Tzu – Old Master.[14] The book is reputedly dated *c.* 550 BCE; certainly from around that time philosophers, recluses and hermits are recorded as living a life devoted to the Tao (the Way of Nature).

However, the second branch of Taoism is of particular interest to us. This is known as Tao Chiao (the Religion of Tao). This also first emerged during the later Han period (*c.* 160 CE). Its founding figures include Chang Tao Ling who lived in the second century CE. Through a combination of dramatic magic and healing, including the use of herbal medicines and elixirs of life, he gained a considerable following. Largely drawn from peasants, his group became one of the main schools of religious Taoism. At around the same time other Taoist religious leaders appeared, combining traditional philosophical ascetic Taoist practices with folk medicine to produce a powerfully attractive new form of popular religion. The old shamanist combination of the supernatural and the natural was at work again. It is important to remember that for every official doctor trained in herbal medicine and using the great texts there were probably ten Taoist priests or adepts who were often illiterate but who practised herbal medicine based upon oral tradition. This thread has continued uninterrupted until this century; indeed, the Communist idea of barefoot doctors owes something to this model. (Interestingly enough, amongst the hundreds of books in the official Taoist canon is found the *Shen-nung Pen Ts'ao Ching*, the pharmaceutical book which is traditionally ascribed to Shen-nung.[15]) So strong was the link between folk medicine and Taoist priests that Buddhist monks, in order to emphasize their separate identity, were forbidden to dabble in medicine unless they were properly trained.

It is appropriate at this stage to examine the very considerable impact which the arrival of Buddhism had upon

herbal medicine. The roots of Buddhism lie in the India of
c. 500 BCE. Arising in opposition to Vedic Hindu teachings, it
nevertheless contained many Vedic ideas and much Indian
knowledge in general. As it moved into China during the first
to the fifth centuries CE it brought with it a whole new world of
belief, thought and practice. The period from c. 55 CE to the
ninth century CE saw a growing intercourse between China and
India as Buddhism slowly took root. Pilgrims, sages, teachers,
translators, trade delegates, ambassadors, texts, etc., crossed
and recrossed the mountains between the two cultures. Part of
this intercourse was directly concerned with healing. India has
long had a profound tradition of herbal medicine. This is
apparent even in her mythology, as, for example, when the
monkey god Hanuman is sent to find herbs to heal the
wounded heroes Rama and Lakshmani.[16] From the second
century CE onwards, Buddhist monks who were accomplished
healers, such as An Shih-kao (second century) and Fo-t'u-teng
(fourth century) appear in the annals. Equally important was
the spread of new ideas and techniques. For instance, Kenneth
Ch'en in his *Buddhism in China* postulates that the celebrated
second-century doctor Hua To may have learned his skills in
surgery from Buddhist accounts of the Indian physician
Jivaka, a contemporary of the Buddha.[17]

By the start of the T'ang dynasty (618 CE) no serious
physician or doctor would not know both the traditional
Chinese texts and the Buddhist texts on medicine. (Witness
the preface to Sun Ssu-miao's classic book *Ch'ien-chin Yao-
fang* (*The Book of Prescriptions Worth a Thousand Gold*) where
he states that to be a great doctor one should read Taoist,
Confucian and Buddhist texts for only thus can one under-
stand the virtues of love, compassion, joy and impartiality.[18]

It is perhaps important to stress that Buddhism also
developed a specifically overt religious side to medicine. Often
in large temples a small room would be set aside for Yun Shi-fo
– the Buddha of Medicine. This is a very popular Buddha who
cures not only worldly sickness but also the sickness of
ignorance. Beside him stand two Bodhisattvas who assist him.
Of particular interest to us is Yao Wang – King of Medicinal
Herbs. (Indeed, the very title of the healing Buddha is best
translated 'the Buddha of Herbal Medicine'.) He is first fully

described in Chinese texts by Hsuan-tsang, the great Chinese
pilgrim to India, *c.* 650 CE and his feast day is the twenty-
eighth day of the fourth month.[19]

Thus, by the time of the T'ang dynasty (*c.* 618–906 CE) the
main streams which have created Chinese herbal medicine had
flowed together.

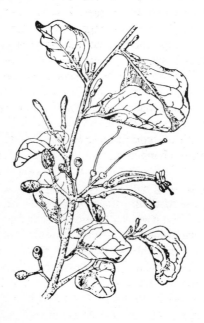

From the T'ang to the late Ming (1368–1644 CE) little of
significance occurred. The known art of herbal medicine was
refined and many books were published, but nothing new of
any great importance took place. It is interesting to note that
the major input of Moslem knowledge during the Mongol
Yuan dynasty (1260–1368) added but a few ideas and herbs to
the stock of Chinese wisdom.

We should, however, pause albeit briefly to acknowledge
the genius of Li Shih-chen (1518–93). Born in Hupei, the area
known as the Province of Medicine, he brought a breath of
fresh air to the herbalist and medical world. Influenced by his
contact with Western scientific and medical works introduced

in translation by the Jesuit fathers, Li Shih-chen produced his work, *Pen Ts'ao Kang Mu* (*The Great Pharmacopoeia*).[20] This laid the foundations for the modern development, and indeed acceptance, of herbal medicine.

The story of herbal medicine runs quietly on until the rise of modernism among China's intellectuals towards the end of the nineteenth century. As part of the traditional Imperial China which they so wished to change, herbal medicine with its religio-magic overtones was regarded as taboo. With the coming of the Republic herbal medicine entered its only period of official scorn, neglect and, in some instances, persecution. This was not the rational scientific medicine which the new men and women of China felt was so vital. So it was relegated to the backwoods and Western medicine was embraced with alacrity.

However, with the coming to power of the Communists in 1949 the situation changed again. Drawn from largely peasant roots, the Communists had lived in poverty alongside the ordinary people long enough to appreciate the undoubted benefits of herbal medicine. Since 1949 medicine in China has sought to 'stand on two legs', namely, to keep the best of traditional Chinese medicine – such as herbal medicine – as well as to make use of the best of Western medicine. It is from the continued use of what many Western doctors have seen as 'old wives' tales' – traditional herbal medicine – by the Communist authorities that the West has only recently become aware of this enormous treasure house of practical knowledge. As recently as 1975 Peter Worsley was able to comment:

In the spirit of self-reliance, the hospitals also manufacture many of the drugs they use, drawing upon traditional pharmacopoeia. In the West much publicity has been given to Chinese use of traditional acupuncture. Much less attention, however, has been paid to the massive use of another traditional resource of Chinese medicine: the pharmacopoeia of drugs that has been the main source of medicines for thousands of years. Today, these are used literally side-by-side with Western drugs: through this door to the clinic, the Western drugs; through that, the dispensing of traditional drugs. I saw some of the raw materials growing on communes, and in the gardens of a Children's Palace. Some of them were familiar, but not familiar friends. To me, they were weeds – dandelions amongst them – I tried hard to eliminate from my garden. Here they were valuable sources of materia medica, from which extracts are made, in the form of powders, pills and liquids, and packed in sanitary ampoules or tubes.[21]

Now, through texts and material made available both by the Chinese themselves and by the practice of Chinese herbal doctors in the West, the tradition is spreading out beyond China. An example of this is the present book. Much of the material comes from Stephen Tang's own family texts and knowledge, accumulated by a family which has records of its ancestors going back thirty-six generations.

Having seen something of its history, we must now turn to look at the concepts which underpin this medicine, concepts utterly different from those upon which Western beliefs about the nature of the body, let alone health, are based.

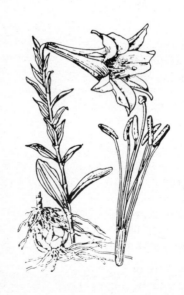

2

THE SCIENCE OF CHINESE HERBAL MEDICINE

The theoretical system upon which Chinese traditional medicine is based represents a different approach to science from that of Western medicine and has its roots in the underlying principles of Chinese culture. The outlines of diagnosis and treatment take into consideration four factors: yin–yang, energy and blood, internal organs and meridians. Medicines are categorized according to:

(i)   the four characteristics – hot, warm, cool, cold;
(ii) the five tastes – sweet, mild, sour, bitter, salt;
(iii) the effect of the medicine within the body, broken down into ascending, descending, floating and sinking;
(iv) the different meridians or channels related to the main organs – the heart, the lungs, the liver, etc.

An essential part of the science of prescribing traditional medicine is called the Harmony of the Seven Sentiments, these being joy, anger, sadness, happiness, worry, pensiveness and fear. These sentiments must be kept in balance in order to keep the body healthy.

Apart from ginseng, which is often used on its own, Chinese herbal medicines are usually given in combination. These combinations are based on a variety of factors.

1. *Complements*   Two or more herbs of similar properties and effects are used together to increase their desired beneficial effects.

2. *Assistants*   Two or more herbs of different properties and effects are used in combination. One herb has the main medicinal effect required, while the other has a catalytic function, increasing the effectiveness of the first herb.

3. *Frights*   One herb is used to moderate the action of another, and thereby to decrease dangerous side effects.

4. *Hates*   One herb is used to modify another's effects so as to achieve the desired result.

5. *Cancellations*   If a herb has inconvenient, though not dangerous, side effects, a second herb may be used to cancel these out.

6. *Contrasts*   This is a miscombination of two herbs and must be avoided at all costs, as it may result in violent bodily reactions and unnecessary side effects.

CAUTIONS

Certain factors must be taken into account as follows:

1.   Consideration must be taken of seasonal, professional and periodic illnesses. If only the individual symptoms are treated, by reference to a handbook, without full consideration of the underlying illness and of the meridian categories of the herbs used, a wrong diagnosis will usually result, leading to complete failure of the treatment.

2.   Special care and attention must be paid to the treatment of pregnant women, since many herbs may induce miscarriage or premature labour, and there is also a slight possibility of damage to the foetus. These herbs are divided into two categories, 'forbidden' and 'careful'; no amateur or inexperienced practitioner should attempt to use them.

3.   When taking Chinese traditional herbal medicine, the patient should bear in mind any advice the doctor may give on food. This will vary according to the condition and the medicines prescribed, but patients are frequently advised to avoid drinking tea while taking herbal medicine.

QUANTITIES

Traditional Chinese herbal medicines are prescribed according to the properties of the particular herbs, their quality and their combination, and the patient's condition, overall health, age, etc., are also taken into account. Certain herbs require carefully laid-down guidelines as to their quantity and ratio: overcautious dosage will not be sufficient to produce the desired effect, while blind overprescription will cause unpleasant and even dangerous results.

There are certain general guidelines which help to determine the constituent elements and quantities of a given medicine.

1. *Category* Elements derived from flowers, hair, skin or leaves are normally prescribed in small amounts. Elements derived from minerals, which are usually dense, are normally prescribed in larger quantities.

2. *Taste* Medicines with little or no taste are prescribed in larger quantities than those with a strong taste.

3. *Combination* The main element in a prescription should be in slightly larger quantities than the others.

4. *Method* If the medicine is to be boiled, then the quantity should be larger than if it is to be made into pills, tablets or a powder.

5. *Condition* The condition of the patient should also determine the quantity; mild cases of an illness need smaller quantities than more serious or extreme cases.

6. *Health* The patient's overall health is important. A normally healthy, active person should receive a higher dosage than a person who was already weak or sickly before the illness.

7. *Age* The very young and the elderly should be given smaller doses than those in the prime of life.

8. *Season* Medicines are prescribed taking into account seasonal changes and their effect on human metabolism.

9. *Environment* Prescriptions also take into account the place where the patient lives/works.

MEDICINAL SOUP

Chinese oral herbal medicines are generally prescribed to be drunk as a soup or a 'tea'. During the boiling process the herbs react chemically, and to achieve the desired results care must be taken over the length of time they are boiled or simmered, and the order in which they are put into the pot; procedures are normally explained by the herbalist to the patient. Patients are frequently advised to avoid drinking tea while taking herbal medicine, since tea itself is regarded as a herbal medicine, being used popularly not only as a pleasant beverage but also for its medicinal effects, which include helping to remove nicotine from the body of smokers. Certain teas are valued for their effects on the activity of the heart, and one of the most popular teas in China is Pu-erh, which is used, among other purposes, to reduce blood sugar and assist weight loss.

Ch'i or Energy

In Chinese medicine Ch'i, or energy, which is a yang force, has two meanings: it is the name for the energy which promotes biological activity; it is also applied to the ability of microscopic material to provide protein.

Overall, Ch'i is the source of growth and disintegration. It is the prime mover and consolidator of the blood, it organizes the whole body, repulses 'evil' attacks from outside the body and promotes the functioning of the internal organs.

More specifically, Ch'i can be broken down into various categories according to its effects upon particular organs.

Original Ch'i   This, which is also known as 'real' or 'correct' Ch'i, represents the body's strength or weakness in combating all forms of illness. When the original Ch'i of a body is restored, illness will be conquered.

Ch'i of Internal Organs   This is the specific energy of particular organs, and so there are the Ch'i of the heart, Ch'i of the liver, Ch'i of the lungs, etc. The Ch'i of the spleen and stomach combined is known as the central Ch'i; if this becomes weakened, it results in difficulties in the functioning of the digestive system, decrease in mental activity, a weak voice and problems with the uterus. These conditions must be treated by a method which strengthens central Ch'i. The Ch'i of the heart and of the lungs together is known as ancestral

Ch'i; this assists respiration and circulation, and its weakening will result in breathing problems and a weak heartbeat.

Guarding Ch'i This is dispersed throughout the body, surrounding all the pulse meridians. It travels outside the meridians and can be regarded as the 'perimeter fence' of all internal systems.

Protein Ch'i This travels within the pulse meridians and provides vital protein to the blood. Guarding Ch'i and protein Ch'i work very closely together.

The disruption of Ch'i can take one of three forms.

1. *Weakening of Ch'i* This means that there is insufficient energy. This is most commonly noticeable when the Ch'i of the lungs and the spleen are weakened; the patent is reluctant to speak and suffers from dizziness, sweating for no apparent reason, loss of appetite and a feeble pulse.

2. *Stagnation of Ch'i* This occurs when the mechanism of internal organ functioning meets an obstruction to its normal operation and is found mainly in the lungs, spleen and liver. It is clearly manifested by tightness in the chest, sides and abdomen, accompanied by pain. Stagnation of Ch'i in the lungs results in tightness of the chest, pain, chestiness in breathing and overproduction of phlegm. If the Ch'i of the spleen is stagnant, it produces a swollen, painful abdomen and indigestion. Stagnation of Ch'i in the liver produces a bloated abdomen, pain in the abdomen, menstrual pain and an irregular menstrual cycle. Stagnation of Ch'i in the meridian veins will result in aching in the joints and muscles of all four limbs.

3. *Mischannelling of Ch'i* This is a flow of energy in the wrong direction. The Ch'i related to each organ in a healthy body travels in a particular direction: for example, the Ch'i of the lungs and of the stomach is supposed to travel downwards. If the flow of Ch'i is in the wrong direction, illness can result. If the lung Ch'i is mischannelled, this causes coughs and asthma; if that of the stomach, vomiting or nausea result; if that of the

liver, the patient experiences fainting, unconsciousness or vomiting of blood.

Blood

Since blood is seen as yin and Ch'i as yang, the two are complementary in their action and equally necessary for health. It is said that 'Ch'i is the ruler of blood, blood is the mother of Ch'i.' The movement of the blood depends on the motivating energy of Ch'i; when Ch'i moves, the blood moves. Stagnation of Ch'i results in clotting of the blood. If there is an insufficient supply of blood, loss of sensitivity and even paralysis can result. Illnesses related to the blood can be divided into three main categories: escape of the blood, weakness of the blood and clotting of blood.

1. *Escape of the Blood*   There are many complex reasons why blood escapes from the various organs of the body; this escape does not, of course, include normal bleeding from superficial cuts caused by minor accidents. Since the causes are so varied, one must first investigate the whole situation to discover the root cause of, for example, vomiting of blood, and the treatment of this may be totally different from that for another form of blood loss, such as excessive menstrual bleeding.

2. *Weakness of the Blood*   Loss of blood in great amounts and the failure of the body's natural ability to manufacture blood also result in weakness of the blood. The concept of blood transfusion is novel to the Chinese, since blood is regarded as something to be treasured. Weakness of the blood results in a distinctive yellowish colour of the skin, pallor of the lips, tongue and nails, dizziness, blurred sight, fainting spells and tiredness; treatment of this condition must be linked with the restoration of Ch'i.

3. *Blood Clotting*   Blood clotting is most commonly seen in the form of bruises, sometimes treated with simple massage or with cold-water massage; nowadays ice is sometimes used, often to very good effect. Clotting of the blood may be caused by external bleeding and can develop in the veins of the heart, lungs or limbs; this can be very painful and may affect

movement. Blood clotting can also be caused by stagnation of Ch'i; if this occurs in the veins of the lungs, it will cause the sufferer to cough up blood.

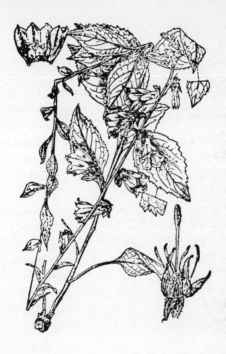

Spirit (Sperm)

'Spirit' is a term with two meanings in Chinese medicine. It can refer to the sperm from which future generations develop; it can also be used for the vital force of cells which is required for human growth. Normally all spirit is stored in the kidneys; part of this becomes sperm.

Dew and Juices

Body fluid is seen in two forms. Dew is the moisture dispersed among the internal organs, muscles and skin; that which is dispersed between the joints and in the brain is known as juices. All body fluids, even sweat and tears, are known as dew or juices.

Dew and blood are seen as closely interrelated: 'Dew and blood are from one source.' Because of this, it was a very early principle of Chinese medicine that those who were prone to loss of blood should not be treated with sudorifics (medicine to produce sweating).

Phlegm is a form of dew. According to Chinese medical theory:

> Spleen is the source of phlegm where it develops,
> Lungs are the reservoir where phlegm is stored.

When excess phlegm is produced in the lungs, as in asthma, it cannot settle properly. Drink is used to combat phlegm, either by expelling or by dispersing it.

Yin and Yang

Chinese medicine uses a simplified version of the theory of two contrasting yet unified forces, yin and yang. Illness is seen to be caused by an imbalance in the relationship of these two forces.

THE ROOTS OF YIN AND YANG

It is said that:

> The beginning of life originates from yin–yang.
> Yin grows from yang, yang grows from yin.
> Yin does not develop on its own, and yet
> Yang does not grow on its own.

In other words, yin and yang are mutually interdependent, and each cannot exist without the other. Without the continued harmony of yin and yang there would be no life.

To take an example from human biology: the abilities of the human body are yang; food is yin. The abilities and power of the body depend on the supply of energy absorbed from food, and yet to obtain that energy the food must be acted upon by the body's functions, such as the digestive system and the circulation of the blood, so as to achieve the desired result, the continuation of life.

EXPANSION AND DIMINUTION OF YIN AND YANG

The theory says that 'When one force expands, the other
diminishes.' The various organs and systems of the human
body are constantly active, and so energy is for ever being
expended and resupplied. This continual process is seen as
normal, but if energy is expended too rapidly, then illness
occurs. For example, there is a type of high blood pressure
which manifests itself in the following symptoms: headache,
dizziness, sleeplessness, short temper and irritability, a dry
red-coloured tongue and a tight pulse which is slower than
normal. This complaint is seen to be caused by a weakening of
yin and a corresponding overexpansion of yang.

The Five Elements

In Chinese philosophy the universe is formed of five basic
elements – gold, wood, water, fire, earth.
   The following table gives a list of correspondences with the
Five Elements:

Element	Wood	Fire	Earth	Gold	Water
Zang internal organs	Liver	Heart	Spleen	Lungs	Kidneys
Fu internal organs	Gall bladder	Small intestine	Stomach	Large intestine	Bladder
Facial features	Eyes	Tongue	Mouth	Nose	Ears
Body	Tendons	Pulse	Muscle	Skin/hair	Bones
Expression	Anger	Gaiety	Thought	Worry	Fright
Colour	Light green	Red	Yellow	White	Black
Taste	Sour	Bitter	Sweet	Pungent	Salt
Energy	Wind	Hot	Wet	Dry	Cold
Season	Spring	Summer	Long summer	Autumn	Winter

The Meridians

The concept of yin and yang is basic to the Chinese idea of the
universe and is important in Chinese medicine. These two
great forces are the source of everything and must be
maintained in balance. Yang, the active force, is seen as male,
associated with the sun, light and fire; while yin, the passive

force, is seen as female, associated with the moon, darkness and water. These forces are seen as being involved in the flow of energy through the body along lines known as meridians. These lines are used by acupuncturists, and can be seen illustrated in acupuncture charts (see diagrams); in acupuncture treatment needles are inserted at several points along a single meridian. In addition, for certain types of pain such as sciatica, another point is used for the insertion of a needle; this does not have a fixed location but is at the point of greatest pain. This point is named after the famous doctor Hua To. Acupuncture seeks to manipulate the flow of energy through the body. For more details of acupuncture, see chapter 7.

Herbal medicine, unlike acupuncture, is concerned with balancing the functioning of the body's organs, which produce all its energy. Yin and yang within the organs must be kept in balance. Although the two approaches are somewhat different,

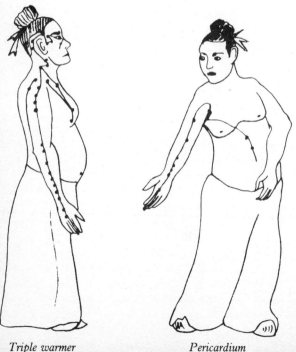

Triple warmer   *Pericardium*

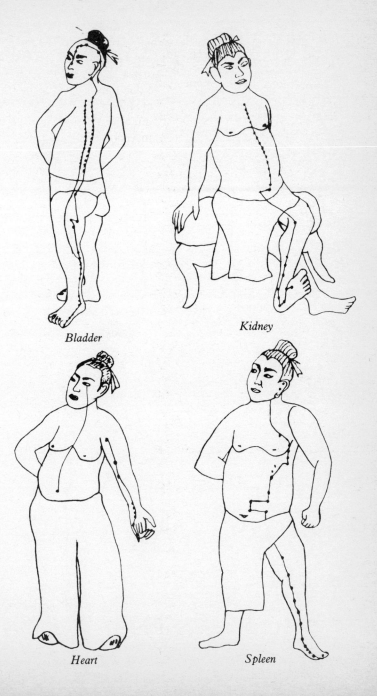

Bladder

Kidney

Heart

Spleen

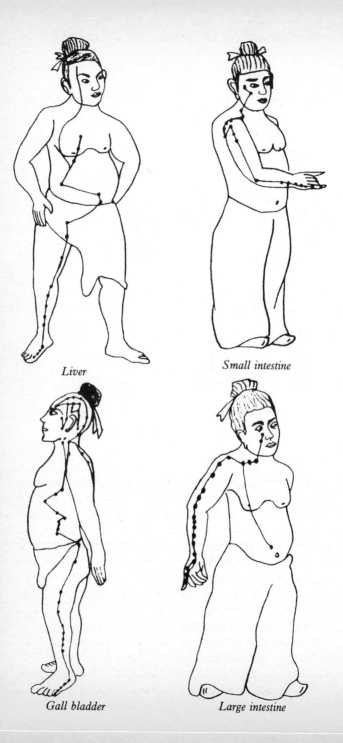

Liver

Small intestine

Gall bladder

Large intestine

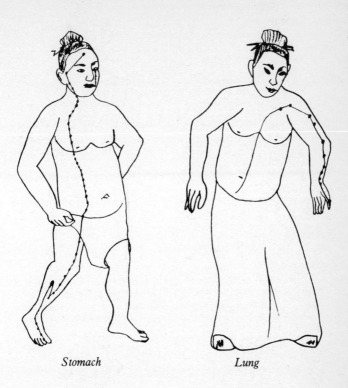

Stomach   Lung

they often work hand in hand. For example, after acupuncture treatment there is often a feeling of immediate relief followed by an intensification of pain; this is the result of stimulation of the nerve points and is to be expected. The use of normal painkillers can interfere with the healing process which has been initiated, so a herbal medicine is usually given; this does not make the pain disappear altogether but makes it bearable. In prolonged illness, acupuncture and herbal medicine are frequently used together. Acupuncture can also be used alongside Western medicine.

All herbs are categorized according to the meridians to which they are related. Herbs associated with different meridians should not be used in combination as this can produce an effect which is the opposite of the one desired, often making the patient worse instead of better.

THE MERIDIAN CHANNELS

The meridian channels can be divided into two categories: real and extra-special channels.

There are twelve pairs of real channels; they are found on both sides of the body and correspond on right and left sides. The three yin channels of hands and of feet and the three yang channels of hands and of feet together make up the twelve Jin Mai or meridians. Each of these meridians is related to a specific internal organ (Zang or Fu); these organs include the Sanjiao or 'triple heaters', which are the three portions of the body cavity.

There are eight extra-special meridians in all, but normally only two of these are used in conjunction with the twelve real meridians, making a total of fourteen Jin Mai.

The twelve real meridians form a complete circulatory system as follows:

Hand (great yin) lung channel → Hand (yang) large intestine channel → Foot (yang) stomach channel → Foot (yin) spleen channel → Hand (yin) heart channel → Hand (yang) small intestine channel → Foot (yang) bladder channel → Foot (yin) kidney channel → Hand (yin) heart/womb channel → Hand (yang) Sanjiao channel → Foot (yang) gall-bladder channel → Foot (yin) liver channel → Hand (great yin) lung channel

Each meridian has associated collateral channels in other parts of the body. These collateral channels are lesser channels linked with the main meridians: the relationship can be visualized as resembling a branching tree, with the meridian as the trunk and its collateral channels as the branches. Every meridian is linked with the treatment of a number of specific complaints. These can be summarized as follows:

THE THREE YIN CHANNELS OF THE HAND

1. *Hand (Great Yin) Lung Channel*   Collateral channels in the large intestine. Used in the treatment of lung, chest and throat complaints.

2. *Hand (Yin) Heart Protected-Wall Channel*   Collateral channels in the Sanjiao. Used to treat heart, stomach and chest complaints, mental deficiency, asthma and diarrhoea.

3. *Hand (Yin) Heart/Womb Channel*   Collateral channels in the small intestine. Used in the treatment of chest diseases, mental disorder and apoplexy.

THE THREE YANG CHANNELS OF THE HAND

1. *Hand (Yang) Large Intestine Channel*   Collateral channels in the lungs. Used in the treatment of complaints of the forehead, face, mouth, teeth, eyes, ears, nose, throat, chest and abdomen, high fever and high blood pressure.

2. *Hand (Yang) Sanjiao Channel* Collateral channels at protected wall of heart. Used in the treatment of complaints of the ears, eyes and throat, and constipation.

3. *Hand (Yang) Small Intestine Channel*   Collateral channel at the heart. Used in the treatment of complaints of the shoulders, neck, head, eyes and throat, mental disorders and high fever.

THE THREE YANG CHANNELS OF THE FOOT

1. *Foot (Yang) Stomach Channel*   Collateral channels at the spleen. Used in the treatment of complaints of the forehead, face, mouth, teeth and throat.

2. *Foot (Yang) Gall-Bladder Channel*   Collateral channels at the liver. Used in the treatment of complaints of the eyes, ears and chest, liver and gall-bladder diseases.

3. *Foot (Yang) Bladder Channel*   Collateral channels at the kidneys. Used in the treatment of complaints of the eyes, top of the skull, back of head, back of the neck and back.

THE THREE YIN CHANNELS OF THE FOOT

1. *Foot (Yin) Spleen Channel* Collateral channels at the stomach. Used in the treatment of stomach diseases, bleeding and loss of sleep.

2. *Foot (Yin) Liver Channel* Collateral channels at the gall bladder. Used in the treatment of illnesses of the liver and the gall bladder.

3. *Foot (Yin) Kidney Channel* Collateral channels at the bladder. Used in the treatment of mental depression.

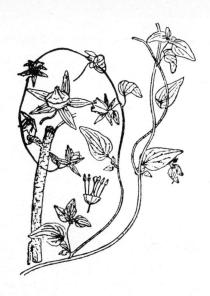

Internal Organs

Zang Fu – internal organs – is an important and integral part of Chinese medical theory. From a holistic viewpoint the human biological system and its activities are seen through the internal organs and the meridians which connect them; all internal organs are dependent on one another, affecting and also restricting one another.

The internal organs are divided into five Zang – heart, liver, spleen, lungs, kidneys – and six Fu (although only five are shown in the preceding table) – stomach, gall bladder, large intestine, small intestine, bladder and Sanjiao (see above).

These are basically similar to Western medical terms, but the correspondence is not exact, so the two sets of terms should not be confused. Differences will be seen in the way the functions of the organs are perceived, as described below.

The five Zang and six Fu work in cooperation, dividing the responsibility for various functions. The five Zang act mainly to preserve and store energy, while the six Fu are responsible in general for sorting out useful from useless substances and for discarding refuse.

HEART AND SMALL INTESTINE

Heart is the master of all internal organs.

1. The heart is the master of spiritual expression, and accordingly is seen as being at the highest level of mental activity. If the function of the heart is in any way impaired, it manifests itself in loss of memory, fear, nervousness, abnormal gestures, etc.

2. As master of the blood and the pulse, the heart cannot be separated from the blood; blood circulation depends on the pumping activity of the heart. The energy of this pump has a direct effect on the circulatory system and so can be detected from the pulse. If the heart's energy is weakened, the pulse feels weak and lacking in strength; if the energy is uneven, the pulse feels irregular and lacking in rhythm.

3. 'Glow in expression, visible on tongue.' The veins on the face and tongue are concentrated, so it can easily be seen from the colour of face and the tongue whether the heart is functioning properly. Even English uses the expression 'radiant' to describe someone who is normal and healthy.

4. 'Sweat is the dew of the heart.' It is important to give careful consideration to the proper administration of medicine whose action involves the production and evaporation of sweat.

5. The heart and small intestine are connected by a meridian and can produce symptoms which are outwardly visible. For example, when 'heartburn heat is diverted to the small intestines' the tip of the tongue may become red and painful.

LIVER AND GALL BLADDER

1. The liver is the master of the movement of energy through the passages in the body. The blockage of energy passages manifests itself, amongst other symptoms, in headaches and menstrual disorder. If yang is too overpowering in the liver, the patient suffers from severe headaches, red and painful eyes, and hearing difficulties.

2.   As master of the blood reserve and of the maintenance of the blood supply, the liver prevents constant bleeding; if it becomes disordered it can result in, for example, vomiting of blood.

3.   The liver and the eyes are closely related. In liver diseases eyesight may be blurred. Many liver complaints are clearly noticeable from the eyes.

4.   As master of tendons, shown in the nails, the liver is the controller of muscles and joints. 'Nails are the extreme ends of muscles'; when the liver blood is healthy the fingernails are red – otherwise the person has difficulty with muscle movements and may even experience convulsions.

5.   The effect of the gall bladder, one of the six Fu, is most recognizable when bitter gall juices are vomited. It is normal practice for the liver and the gall bladder to be treated together.

From the above we can see that the Chinese physiology and pathology of the liver and the gall bladder basically correspond to those of Western theory, but also include the blood circulation system and eyesight.

SPLEEN AND STOMACH

1.   The spleen is the master of the circulatory systems and the organ of energy absorption. When the spleen is working normally the stomach functions properly and the person is full of vitality.

2.   The spleen is also the warden of the blood and is believed to be the manufacturer of the blood.

3.   It is the controller of the muscles in hands and feet and its action is detectable from the lips. A weakened spleen affects the appetite, causing thinness (as opposed to slimness), lack of strength in hands and feet, with the lips becoming white, pale or yellow.

4.   The stomach is the ocean of liquid or food. The Chinese say that 'The energy of the stomach is the vital energy of life', whereas the spleen is the fundamental restorer after birth. The

spleen is therefore yin and the stomach is yang. Stomach disorders can produce toothache.

From the above it can be seen that while the Chinese concept of the stomach is close to the Western concept, that of the spleen is quite different from the Western idea.

LUNGS AND LARGE INTESTINE

1.   Chinese see the lungs as the master of Ch'i to all internal organs as well as to all the meridians. Disorder in their functioning will result in asthma, shortness of breath, a weak, low voice, and a lack of patience in explaining things because the person becomes too lazy to speak.

2.   The liver is the master of passage, which includes the flow of both air and water in the body. Ch'i in the lungs is so necessary even for the passing of water that it is said that the lungs are 'the origin of water above'.

3.   The action of the lungs is visible in the nose, since this is where air enters. This is one of the more obvious signs of the lungs' functioning. The lungs, the ability to speak and the level of sound are also closely connected; in extreme cases the voice may be lost.

4.   The large intestine and the lungs are seen to be connected in function because they are both needed to provide passage.

KIDNEYS AND BLADDER

1.   As master of sperm (spirit), the role of the kidneys is, first, to preserve the spirit of the reproductive system and, secondly, to preserve the vital spirits of all the body's organs. The treatment of any reproductive disorder is always concentrated on the kidneys.

2.   The kidneys are seen as the organ of water, and are implicated if one passes water too frequently or has to get up several times during the night to urinate.

3.   The kidneys are master of bone, marrow and brain. Kidney weakness causes slowness in movement and, in

children, hinders the development of intelligence. Also, since 'teeth are the end of the bones', kidney problems result in loss of teeth.

4. Although the kidneys are seen as the organ of water, they are also known as 'the fire at the gate of life'. Kidney yang is vital to human existence: kidney spirit and water are yang. If the fire at the gate of life is weak, impotence and premature ejaculation result; if it is too strong, it can result in sexual overindulgence and irritability during the day.

5. Hearing problems and constipation can be caused by kidney disorder.

6. The normal and abnormal functioning of the kidneys can be seen in the hair: weak kidneys cause loss or greying of the hair.

7. The bladder is seen as related to the kidneys because of the close cooperation of their functions.

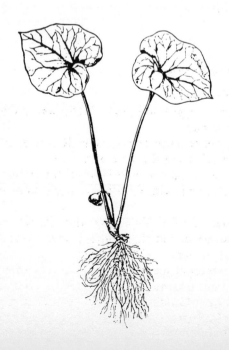

THE THREE CONCENTRATIONS

The body is divided into three areas: upper, middle and lower. Upper consists of heart and lungs and roughly corresponds to the chest. Middle consists of the spleen and stomach; lower, the liver, kidneys, bladder and intestine. Their roles are seen as: upper – receiving; middle – transporting; lower – passing or rejecting.

THE WOMB

Applicable only of course to the female, this affects the female cycle, pregnancy and the reproductive system.

The Relationship and Functions of the Internal Organs (Zang Fu)

The internal organs are divided into Zang, Fu and special permanent Fu.

FIVE ZANG

Combined Ability   Preservation of energy (Ch'i).

Individual Functions
Heart: Master of spirit and pulse. Condition visible from the state of the tongue.
Liver: Master of passages and tendons. Reservoir of the blood. Condition visible from the state of the eyes.
Spleen: Master of the circulatory systems. Commander of the blood, muscles and skin. Condition visible from the state of the mouth.
Lungs: Master of Ch'i, air and energy. Forces clearance of passages. Master of the skin and the hair. Condition visible from the state of the nose.
Kidneys: Preserver of sperm (spirit). Master of water and bone. Provider of bone marrow, which includes the brain. Master of fire at life's gate. Condition visible from the state of the ears and the private parts.

SIX FU

Combined Ability   Reception, digestion, transmission and passage.

Individual Functions
Stomach: Receiver of water and foodstuff.
Small intestine: Digestion and reception of foodstuff. Separation of different forms of energy usage.
Large intestine: Passing of wastes.
Bladder: Reservoir and passer of urine.
Sanjiao: Transport of liquid and foodstuff. Passing of wastes.
Gall bladder: Preservation of gall juice.

SPECIAL PERMANENT FU

Combined Ability   Conservation of energy (Ch'i).

Individual Functions
Brain: Mental command. Controls functions.
Marrow: Provision of bone.
Bone: Gives structure to the body.
Veins (pulse): Circulation of the blood.
Womb: Provides female menstrual and reproductive cycle.

Diagnosis

The precise diagnosis of a patient's problem is not a simple matter. A Western doctor may be content to say that a patient has influenza, but a Chinese doctor will wish to know whether the influenza is hot or cold, wet or dry, upward-floating or sinking. Even sweat can be hot or cold.

One of the methods sometimes used for arriving at a diagnosis is the tasting of the patient's sweat. From the taste of the sweat an experienced Chinese doctor can tell a great deal about the condition of the patient. The sweat may be tasteless, salty or sour, and this gives more information about the illness. Because the sense of taste is so important to the doctor, he must cleanse his mouth before a consultation; smokers are, of course, at a disadvantage and if a doctor smokes he must refrain from doing so while examining patients if he is using this technique.

Another diagnostic method, more familiar to the Westerner, is the examination of the pulse. The speed of the pulse is important, as is its strength: it may be so strong that no pressure is required to feel it or so weak that it can hardly be felt at all.

The overall demeanour of the patient can give strong indications about his health and state of mind: an exhausted person moves quite differently from someone in a tense, irritable frame of mind.

The precision of diagnosis is vital for the accurate prescription of herbal medicine. For example, if a patient is suffering from a cold sweat, it is extremely inadvisable to prescribe a cooling herb.

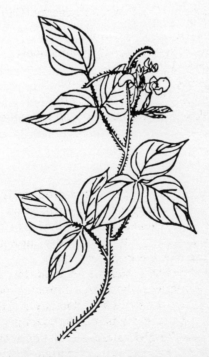

3

PREPARATION AND PROPERTIES OF HERBS

The relationship between the Chinese doctor and the herbalist, although in some ways similar to that between the Western doctor and the pharmacist, differs in some important respects. There are two main types of doctor using traditional herbal medicine, both equally respected for their knowledge and skills: those who are textbook trained and those who are trained through practice and experience. The former have little or no experience of fresh herbs and will recognize them only in their prepared form; the latter know a great deal about herbs in their raw as well as their prepared forms. The herbalist, however, knows more about herbs than both. An experienced herbalist will have acquired enough skill in diagnosis to supply remedies for a large number of ailments and to check patients for possible side effects of medication, although his ability in this field is not as great as that of the trained doctor. His knowledge of herbs enables him to substitute herbs of similar effect for any in the prescription which are for some reason unavailable or are particularly expensive. This knowledge was even more important in the past, when doctors usually travelled great distances and herbs were not frequently exported from one area to another: the herbalist could replace the herbs in the doctor's personal repertoire with locally grown equivalents. Another problem which herbalists used to encounter was that those who had little money often had to save up for some time to pay for the medicine; of course, by the time they had done so the illness might well be at a different stage. A wise herbalist would always check the date on the prescription and, if necessary, change the ingredients or quantities to suit the patient's new needs.

A good herbalist needs to be not only an accomplished botanist but also a very good mountaineer, since the best herbs for medicine are those growing in an undisturbed environment as far from human habitation as possible. The quality of herbs also varies according to region and to the season in which they are picked. When gathering plants the herbalist makes it a rule not to take the whole plant unless absolutely necessary, and at any rate to leave some specimens of that particular herb still growing so that they can be returned to later.

Once herbs are gathered they need to be treated to preserve their qualities for storage. They are always washed and dried, but the precise method of drying can vary; they may be sun-dried or dried in a clay oven, alone or with other herbs. Sometimes they are dried with minerals such as sulphur, which bleaches them and also acts as a preservative.

Herbs are sometimes referred to as 'treated'. This means that, after drying, they are stir-fried with angelica and milk vetch to enhance their properties. Some may also be buried in the ground to absorb moisture or cooked in a clay pot with rice wine or honey, which makes them more powerful.

Either before or after this treatment, the herb is cut up in one of several different ways. Large roots are often sliced across at 90 degrees, which gives a round cross-section, while smaller plants are cut at an angle to give a larger surface area. Some herbs are chopped very finely and compressed into a cake. Traditionally, these herbs are then stored in clay pots, the shape of which and whether they are covered or uncovered depending on the herb. Nowadays glass bottles are often used for storage. In a herbalist's shop the herbs are generally kept in drawers for convenience of dispensing. An experienced herbalist is expected not to label these drawers; he or she should be totally familiar with their contents. Since the drawers are arranged according to meridians, properties and so forth, a mistake by the herbalist will not have an adverse effect. This system of arrangement is also useful if one herb needs to be substituted for another.

However the herbs are stored, the herbalist must check them periodically for mould or other signs of deterioration, since if these checks are not made the whole stock is endangered. Herbs may need to be retreated, that is washed

and boiled, redried and, where necessary, treated with angelica, etc., just as for fresh herbs.

When a herbalist fills out a prescription, which is normally
for three doses of medicine, he or she works in a particular
way, setting out each ingredient individually on a sheet of
paper. This enables the ingredients to be checked against the
prescription when they have all been weighed out. At busy
times the herbalist and an assistant may fill out a prescription
together, working from opposite ends towards the middle.
When seeds are prescribed, they are usually ground using a
mortar and pestle, and it is said that one can tell the experience
of a herbalist from the sound of the mortar and pestle as he or
she uses them.

The herbalist will select herbs of a particular quality
according to a patient's means. Different grades of herbs are
common; for example, angelica from some areas of China is

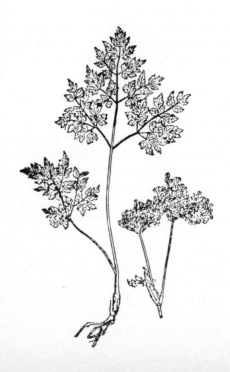

much less highly regarded than that from other areas. One of
the herbs most often graded in this way is ginseng. Because it
is so expensive, this herb is weighed in very sensitive scales,
which have divisions of 0·1 g. Other herbs do not need quite
such accurate scales. Whichever scales are used, the weight
given in prescriptions is always that of the herb before any stir-
frying which is called for by the prescription, whether the herb
is to be fried in honey, in water, or in rice wine, or 'burned'
until black in a red-hot wok. Since these treatments change the
weight of the herb, it is not unknown for patients to weigh
their herbs afterwards and mistakenly complain that they have
been short-changed by the herbalist.

Implements

A wide variety of implements are used in Chinese herbal
medicine, both in preparing herbs in their raw state and in
preparing medicines from the herbs. In general their materials
and construction have remained the same for hundreds of
years, although modern versions may be used if they are as
effective. Those illustrated here are among the most commonly used.

Chinese scales for weighing herbs come in two sizes. The
larger scales are used for weighing ordinary herbs and are
accurate to within approximately 3 g, while the smaller scales
are used for more precious and expensive ingredients such as
ginseng. Both sorts of scales are used by holding one of the
strings near the pan and adjusting the weight on the rod.

For the convenience of the Western reader, we have used
metric weights in the present book. The herbalist will, of
course, use Chinese weights. These are as follows:

1 fan		= 0·3 g approx.
10 fan	= 1 qin	= 3 g approx.
10 qin	= 1 lian	= 30 g approx.
16 lian	= 1 jin	= 480 g approx.

Often herbs need to be ground to a powder, and this is done
using a mortar and pestle. The mortar has a lid to avoid the
loss of powder during crushing.

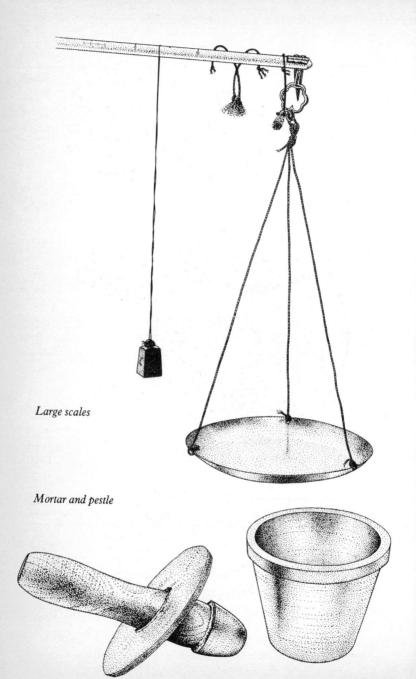

Large scales

Mortar and pestle

Steam pot

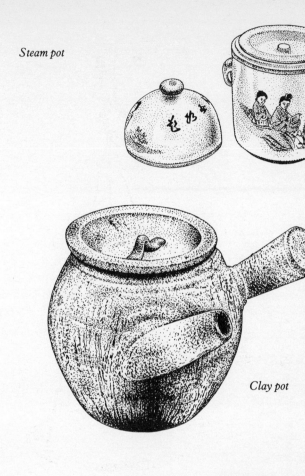

Clay pot

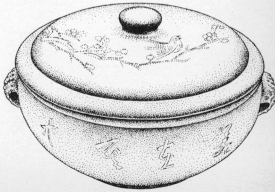

Decorated pot

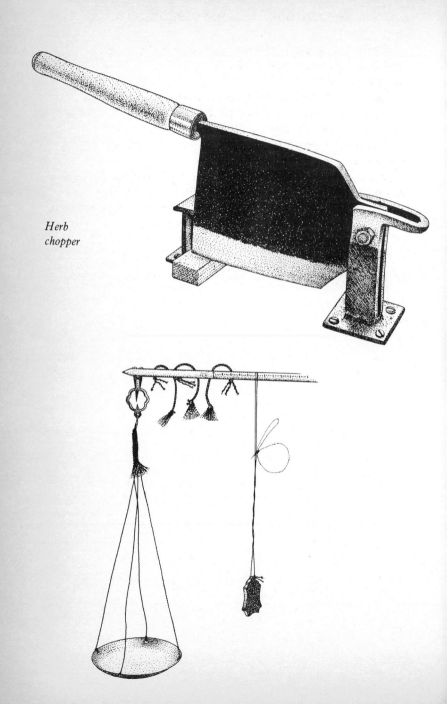

*Herb
chopper*

When herbs need to be chopped, this is done using a guillotine-like implement which can cope with the thickest and toughest of roots.

Herbs are boiled in a clay pot; these come in a variety of sizes. It used to be a tradition to throw all used medicine pots away on the eve of Chinese New Year; however, herbalists in the West can rarely afford to throw away such a comparatively expensive piece of equipment.

Steam pots are used particularly for medicinal food (see pp. 96–101). The ingredients are put into the pot (these again come in several sizes), both lids are put on and fastened by a string which passes through the handles and the pot is placed in a larger pot of boiling water. The herbs and other ingredients are cooked by the rising steam without losing any valuable elements which might be boiled out.

4

SPECIFIC HERBS

It would be impossible to describe all the herbs used in Chinese medicine in the short space available. The following are a few of the most useful and widely used.

Acorus gramineus

Part used: root
Meridians: heart, spleen, stomach
Taste: tangy

For excess of phlegm and delirium, the herb is used with Cape jasmine (*Gardenia jasminoides*), young bamboo leaves and extracted ginger juice. To treat tinnitus and amnesia, it is given with Indian bread (*Poria cocos*) and milkwort (*Polygala sibirica*). For loss of appetite, it is taken with *Agastache rugosus*, magnolia (*Magnolia officinalis*) and tangerine peel.

Dosage: 3–9 g

Artemisia annua, A. apiacea

Part used: leaves
Meridians: liver, gall bladder
Taste: bitter

Fresh leaves of artemisia, crushed and applied externally, are used in the treatment of burns and minor skin diseases. The herb is also used in the treatment of malaria, in combination with skullcap (*Scutellaria baicalensis*), *Pinellia ternata* and arrowroot. This herb has a very pleasant smell.

Dosage: 6–15 g (20–40 g for malaria)

Note: This herb does not require lengthy boiling.

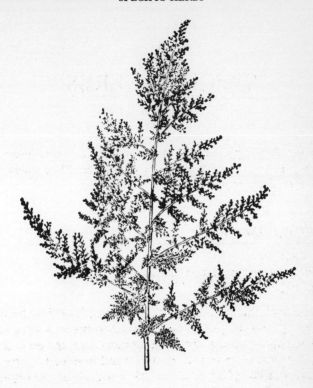

Artemisia apiacea

Asparagus cochinchinensis

Part used: root
Meridians: lungs, kidneys
Taste: bitter-sweet

This herb is used raw and sliced. It is a restorer of yin; it dispels heat and strengthens the lungs and kidneys. To treat a dry cough with very little sputum or coughing up of blood, use it with *Ophiopogon japonicus* and fritillary bulb (*Fritillaria verticillata*). Use this herb in the treatment of whooping cough, assisted by *Ophiopogon japonicus* and stemona root (*Stemona sessilifolia*).

Dosage: 6–12 g

Atractylis macrocephala

Part used: root
Meridians: spleen, stomach
Taste: bitter-sweet

This herb is used to correct mischannelling of Ch'i at the spleen and stomach. It is used to treat loss of appetite, fullness or tightness of the abdomen, vomiting and bowel disorders. It can be used during pregnancy.

Dosage: 4·5–9 g

Barrenwort (*Epimedium brevicornu, E. koreanum, E. sagittatum*)

Part used: the whole plant apart from the root
Meridians: liver, kidneys
Taste: sweet

This herb is used to treat impotence, paralysis of the lower limbs and high blood pressure in elderly women.

Dosage: 3–9 g

Cinnamon (*Cinnamomum cassia*)

Part used: bark
Meridians: heart, lungs, bladder

If the patient sweats, cinnamon is given in combination with peeled peony. If the patient is not sweating, it is given in combination with ma huang (*Ephedra sinica*). Used in combination with various herbs such as *Stenocoelium divaricatum*, *Notopterygium incisum* and *Aconitum balfourii* or *A. chinense* to relieve pain in the joints. Combined with herbs such as Chinese angelica (*Angelica sinensis*) or *Ligustrum wallichii*, this herb is used to treat period pains and menstrual irregularity.

Dosage: 3–9 g (slightly more if used for arthritis)

Note: Should be avoided during pregnancy.

Phellopterus littoralis

Part used: root
Meridians: lungs, stomach
Taste: bitter-sweet

This herb restores yin. For the treatment of coughs it is used with *Ophiopogon japonicus* and mulberry leaves (*Morus alba*).

Dosage: 4·5–9 g

Cornelian cherry (*Cornus officinalis*)

Part used: flesh of fruit
Meridians: liver, kidneys
Taste: bitter, sour

This herb is used in the treatment of abnormally heavy menstruation, and is also used with ginseng to treat heavy sweating accompanied by extreme exhaustion.

Dosage: 4·5–9 g

Cuscuta chinensis

Part used: seeds (boiled and crushed, sometimes in cake form)
Meridians: lungs, kidneys
Taste: sweet

Used to treat lack of yang in the kidneys, which causes frequent urination; this herb is also used to prevent miscarriages. It is given with other herbs of similar properties to restore the functions of the kidneys and the menstrual cycle.

Dosage: 6–12 g

Gastrodia elata

Part used: tuber
Meridian: liver
Taste: sweet

When used to clear collateral channels and to relieve pain caused by rheumatism, it is taken with *Lonicera parasitica*,

Achyranthes bidentata and/or Chinese angelica (*Angelica sinensis*). For migraine, dizziness and eyesight disorders, it is used with *Pinellia ternata*, *Atractylis macrocephala*, and/or Indian bread (*Poria cocos*). Commonly used by women suffering from headaches, especially after childbirth.

Dosage: 3–9 g boiled in water
       1–1·5 g as a powder

Liquorice (*Glycyrrhiza glabra, G. uralensis, G. inflata*)

Part used: root
Meridians: all
Taste: sweet

This is one of the most frequently used herbs in Chinese medicine. It can be used on its own to assist the spleen, restore Ch'i, dispel heat and treat sore throats and food poisoning. It is also used to relieve any discomfort which may be felt after taking other medicinal herbs. It is, however, most often used with other herbs to mediate their effects.

Dosage: 1·5–9 g

Lycium barbarum

Part used: seed
Meridians: liver, kidneys
Taste: sweet

If used for weakness of liver or kidneys, dizziness, tinnitus or weakness of the knees or for the prevention of wet dreams, it is taken with *Rehmannia glutinosa* and *Asparagus cochinchinensis*. To strengthen the spirit and the kidneys and to improve eyesight, it is prescribed with *Rehmannia glutinosa*, chrysanthemum (*Chrysanthemum morifolium*) and cornelian cherry (*Cornus officinalis*).

Dosage: 6–12 g

Magnolia liliflora

Part used: flower
Meridians: none specific
Taste: tangy

Clears running nose and headaches; used for the treatment of rhinitis and nasosinusitis.

Dosage: 1–3 g

Ma Huang (*Ephedra sinica*)

Part used: stalk
Meridians: lungs, bladder
Taste: tangy

Always use in combination with cinnamon to aid sweating. To restore the function of the lungs and suppress asthma linked with coughing, it is usually stir-fried in honey and commonly combined with apricot kernels (*Prunus armeniaca*). To reduce swelling, it is usually used in combination with fresh ginger and *Atractylis macrocephala*.

Dosage: 3–9 g

Note: Not suitable for patients who are already sweating or suffering from insomnia or high blood pressure.

Milk Vetch (*Astragalus membranaceus*)

Part used: root
Meridians: spleen, lungs
Taste: sweet

This herb is used sliced, either raw or stir-fried in honey. It is given as a tonic to those debilitated by illness or feeling generally weak and tired and is often prescribed in conjunction with ginseng. Symptoms which indicate the use of this herb include shortness of breath, coldness, loss of appetite and a tendency to sweat easily. It is one of the most commonly prescribed herbs in Chinese medicine.

Dosage: 9–30 g

Milkwort (*Polygala sibirica*)

Part used: root (chopped into sections and treated with liquorice)
Meridians: heart, kidneys, lungs
Taste: bitter

This herb is used to treat depression, irritability and insomnia.

Dosage: 3–9 g

Ophiopogon japonicus

Part used: root nodules
Meridians: lungs, heart, stomach
Taste: bitter-sweet

This herb restores yin. It is used raw and pressed flat. For coughs or dry throats, it is combined with *Pinellia ternata*, *Campanumoea pilosula* and liquorice. For insomnia, it is given with *Rehmannia glutinosa*, figwort (*Scrophularia nodosa*), golden thread (*Coptis chinensis*) and *Salvia multiorrhiza*.

Dosage: 6–12 g

Peony (*Paeonia lactiflora, P. obovata, P. veitchii*)

Part used: root
Meridian: liver
Taste: sweet

This herb is used in chopped slices, together with Chinese angelica (*Angelica sinensis*), *Ligustrum wallichii* and safflower (*Carthamus tinctorius*), for abdominal pains after childbirth.

Dosage: 6–15 g

Note: Do not use with black false hellebore.

Perilla frutescens

Part used: leaves
Meridians: lungs, spleen
Taste: sweet

This herb promotes Ch'i; it is usually used to treat pain and tightness in the abdomen, food poisoning (especially that caused by seafood), vomiting and diarrhoea.

Dosage: 6–12 g

Rehmannia glutinosa

Part used: root (fresh or oven-dried)
Meridians: heart, liver, kidneys
Taste: sweet

Used to counter coldness in the blood. For high body temperature, with a dry mouth and red tongue, the herb is used with figwort (Scrophularia ningpoensis). It is given with lotus leaves and Rubia cordifolia for blood in vomit or urine. For a macula or dark spot on the skin, it is used with the bark of tree peony (Paeonia suffruticosa). To treat thirst associated with diabetes, it is given with Chinese yam (Dioscorea batatas) and Chinese wolfberry (Lycium chinense).

Dosage: 9–30 g (double if fresh)

Treated   (dried, then fried in rice wine until dark)

Meridians: heart, liver, kidneys

Used for restoration of the blood, tinnitus, weakness of the knees and menstrual disorders.

Dosage: 9–15 g

Sanchi (Gynura pinnatifida)

Part used: whole plant
Meridians: liver, kidneys
Taste: bitter

This herb is also known as tienchi and is similar to ginseng. It disperses bruises, arrests haemorrhaging and relieves swellings and pain.

Dosage: for wounds and pains 1–1.5 g powder three times a
   day
for cardiac arrest 1·5 g twice a day in equal proportions with
   ginseng

Schizandra chinensis, S. sphenanthera

Part used: fruit
Meridians: lungs, heart, kidneys
Taste: sour

The two forms of this plant used in Chinese herbal medicine are commonly known as the northern plant (*S. chinensis*) and the southern plant (*S. sphenanthera*). The Chinese name for the herb means 'the seed (or fruit) which has five tastes'. It can be used raw or steamed with vinegar or rice wine. It is used for coughs caused by weakness of the lungs, sometimes in combination with ginseng. It is also used with *Ophiopogon japonicus* to treat patients who sweat, tire easily, have a dry mouth and are depressed.

Dosage: 1·5–6 g

Schizonepeta tenuifolia

Part used: seeds
Meridians: none specific
Taste: tangy

This herb is used to stop swellings and is a good painkiller; it is one of the main herbs used in the treatment of arthritis. Fried until very dark in colour, it is used to stop bleeding, especially from haemorrhoids.

Dosage: 3–9 g

Skullcap (*Scutellaria baicalensis*)

Part used: root
Meridians: lungs, large intestine, small intestine, spleen,
  gall bladder
Taste: bitter

This herb can be used raw, sliced or stir-fried in rice wine. For pain in the throat, it is used with weeping forsythia (*Forsythia suspensa*) and honeysuckle. For high blood pressure, it is used with chrysanthemum and *Nauclea rhynchophylla*.

Dosage: 3–10 g

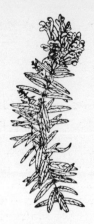

*Scutellaria
baicalensis*

Tree Peony (*Paeonia suffruticosa*)

Part used: bark
Meridians: heart, liver, kidneys
Taste: bitter

To stimulate the manufacture of blood and to disperse bruises, the herb is used fried in rice wine. For period pain, it is used in raw slices. In both cases it is given with cinnamon and walnuts. To stop bleeding in internal wounds, it is dry-fried until dark and given with safflower. For menstrual disorders, it is used with *Bupleurum chinense* and Chinese angelica (*Angelica sinensis*). In cases of high blood pressure, it is used with chrysanthemum (*Chrysanthemum morifolium*) and honeysuckle stem.

Dosage: 6–12 g

Note: Not suitable for use during pregnancy.

Tsi (*Houttuynia cordata*)

Part used: whole herb
Meridians: lungs, kidneys
Taste: sweet

Also known as fishes' smell plant, it has a fishy odour. Used for the treatment of lung- and kidney-related diseases.

Dosage: 9–30 g

Nauclea rhynchophylla (also *Uncaria macrophylla, U. sessilifructus*)

Part used: thorn
Meridians: liver, heart
Taste: sweet

To stop convulsions, spasms and tics, this herb is given with *Gastrodia elata*. For the treatment of reddened eyes caused by headache, it is prescribed together with chrysanthemum (*Chrysanthemum morifolium*), mulberry leaves (*Morus alba*) and menthol. It does not need boiling.

Dosage: 6–12 g

Wikstroemia indica

Part used: roots, leaves
Meridians: none specific
Taste: bitter

Used to reduce swelling and to treat asthma and whooping cough. This herb can be taken orally, but because of its poisonous nature it should be given in extremely small doses and boiled for at least three hours to reduce its toxicity. The leaves can be used externally, crushed and applied to the skin and wrapped well in bandages.

Note: Treat with extreme caution.

Herbs for Common Ailments

The following are a selection of some of the herbs most frequently used for treatment of colds and flu, coughs and sore eyes.

FOR INFLUENZA AND COLDS

Mulberry leaves (*Morus alba*)	6–12 g
Muscadine grape (*Vitex rotundifolia*)	3–10 g
Plantain, whole herb (*Plantago major*)	15–30 g
Plantain, seed (*Plantago major*)	3–10 g

Cape jasmine (*Gardenia jasminoides*)	3–9 g
Balloon flower (*Platycodon grandiflorus*)	3–10 g

TO TREAT COUGHS

Mulberry leaves (*Morus alba*)	6–12 g
Glehnia littoralis	10–15 g
Mint (*Mentha arvensis*)	6 g
Plantain, whole herb (*Plantago major*)	15–30 g
Plantain, seed (*Plantago major*)	3–10 g
Balloon flower (*Platycodon grandiflorus*)	3–10 g
Pat ho (*Lilium brownii*)	30–60 g

FOR SORE EYES

Mulberry leaves (*Morus alba*)	6–12 g
Muscadine grape (*Vitex rotundifolia*)	3–10 g
Chrysanthemum (*Chrysanthemum indicum*)	3–10 g

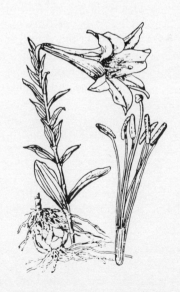

Lilium brownii

CHINESE HERBAL PRESCRIPTIONS

Chinese prescriptions fall into several categories. (In the following descriptions the numbers refer to individual prescriptions – see pp. 73–95.)

SWEAT-EVAPORATION METHOD

Prescriptions of this type have several purposes:

(a) To promote sweating. This helps to dispel certain cold-related symptoms: high fever, stuffy or running nose, headache, general pain all over the body, white tongue and floating pulse.

   This group can be further divided into extension-of-warmth and extension-of-cold methods. The former are used to treat illnesses with cold-related symptoms and include Ma Huang Soup (1) and Cinnamon Soup (2). The latter are used to treat illnesses with heat-related symptoms and include Honeysuckle and Forsythia Powder (3) and Mulberry and Chrysanthemum Drink (4).

(b) To assist the rapid development and disappearance of rashes in, for example, the early stages of chickenpox. Prescriptions used for this include Cimicifuga and Pueraria Soup (5).

(c) To remove wetness through evaporation of sweat. These prescriptions are used to treat cold-winded and wetness-related diseases, typical symptoms of which are enlargement of the head, heaviness of the body, pain, a white tongue, floating, slow pulse and an outward appearance of wetness. Such prescriptions include Ma Huang and Cinnamon Soup (6).

(d) To relieve swelling. This is achieved by evaporation, which not only disperses wetness through sweating but also clears the lung passages of Ch'i. These prescriptions cause the concentrated fluids to be transported to the bladder, promote the passing of wind and relieve swelling. They include Yer Pi Soup (7) and the Prescription to Expel Wind and Promote the Passage of Water (8), and are used to treat yang water illnesses, which manifest themselves in a swollen body with wind and a floating pulse.

The above prescriptions, through sweating, also cause expansion in the veins, increased circulation of the blood and an increase in the heat escaping from the body which causes lowering of the temperature. They are often used to treat influenza and are also widely prescribed for loss of voice, infected tonsils, bronchitis, lung infections, mumps and measles. They are used in conjunction with Western medicine in the treatment of allergies, kidney problems and acute rheumatism, to increase the effectiveness of the treatments and promote recovery after the illness.

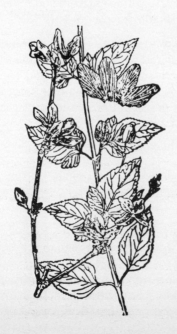

LOWER-FLOWING PRESCRIPTIONS

Also known as the downward method, these prescriptions are laxative and dispel hotness and water.

Lower-flowing prescriptions are divided into several groups according to the different forms of symptoms treated, their origins and whether the medicine is required to act quickly or slowly.

(a)   Cool lower flow. These are used to treat those who are solid and hot internally, with hard stools, bloated abdomen, pain, high temperature, thirst, headache, delirium, vomiting of blood and stagnation of the energy in the internal organs. Prescriptions used include Da Zheng Qi Soup (9) and Lian Gor Powder (10).

(b)   Warm lower flow. These are used to treat emptiness, weakness and a gathering of cold in the spleen, accompanied by hardness of the bowels, coldness in the limbs and a sinking, slow pulse, or to treat concentrated yin cold which shows itself in expansion of the bowels, oedema or dropsy and difficulty in passing stools. Prescriptions used include Warm Spleen Soup (11) and Rhubarb and Aconitum Soup (12).

(c)   Moist downward flow. These are used to treat an overconcentration of whatever is affecting the fluid (dew), symptoms of dryness after illness or owing to old age, symptoms of weakness in the blood affecting the bowels after childbirth, and long-standing hardness of bowel movement. Prescriptions used include Wu Yan Pills (13).

(d)   Dispelling of water. These prescriptions are used to treat fluids which gather in the body or moisture concentrated in the chest, swollen abdomen, stagnation of Ch'i in the internal organs and a yellow tongue. Prescriptions include Ten Jujube Soup (14).

(e)   Cold lower flow. These prescriptions activate the large intestine. They are used as antibiotics, antiseptics, neutralizing agents and in the treatment of diarrhoea. They are prescribed to control allergies in their active stage, and also for lung infections and a variety of more serious complaints. They are also suitable for use with symptoms of high fever, thirst, constipation, full and painful abdomen and delirium. They are used in cases of acute conjunctivitis, nosebleeds or high blood pressure which are associated with headaches. Over the past twenty years they have commonly been used for acute appendicitis, liver disease and chronic constipation.

Apart from the moist downward-flow prescriptions, these prescriptions should not be taken over a long period.

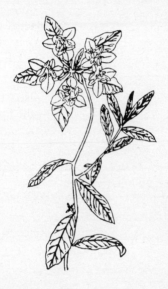

MEDIATING PRESCRIPTIONS

These use mild and moderately strong forms to treat symptoms which are half external and half internal, disharmony of the liver and spleen and other similar problems.

The peculiar characteristic of this group of prescriptions is their combination of warmth and cold, attack and preservation, to achieve a balance between the external and the internal. They aim to achieve a harmony between yin and yang and between all the internal organs.

(a) Mediation of half external and half internal symptoms. The symptoms are fluctuating heat and coldness, fullness in the chest, loss of appetite, a bitter taste in the mouth, dry throat and dizziness. It is difficult to treat these with medicines which only cause sweating or lower the flow, so it is necessary to use a mediating treatment such as Bupleurum Tonic (15).

(b) Mediation of the spleen and the liver. In cases of stagnation of Ch'i in the liver or tiredness of the spleen and stomach, the following symptoms may be experienced: bloating of the chest and waist, loss of appetite, bowel disorders, loss of spirit, and disharmony between the liver and the spleen and between the liver and the stomach. When these symptoms are experienced, prescriptions which mediate between the spleen and the liver are used: these include Chao Yan Powder (16), Zi Yi Tonic (17) and Pain and Diarrhoea Prescription (18).

(c) Mediation of the stomach and the intestine. These prescriptions are used in cases of an imbalance between heat or warmth and cold, and disorders of the stomach and intestine. Symptoms which are experienced include a concentration of heat and a feeling of nausea without actual vomiting, along with a pain in the abdomen which is caused by a concentration of cold in the intestine. An example of prescriptions of this type is Huang Lian Soup (19).

(d) Mediation and treatment of malaria. Malaria is seen as an illness which is half internal and half external; its symptoms include fluctuations between heat and cold, fullness at the chest and waist and a feeling of nausea without actual vomiting. Prescriptions used in the treatment of this illness include Bupleurum Tonic (15) and Seven Wonder Tonic (20). It may be necessary in individual cases to add or subtract one or two of the ingredients from either of these prescriptions.

Mediating prescriptions form the most widely used group of prescriptions in Chinese traditional medicine.

INTERNAL-WARMTH PRESCRIPTIONS

These are also known as the 'cold dispelling method'. Prescriptions of this type use herbs with warming or heating properties to remove and replace internal cold, to treat cold which has concentrated in the meridians and internal organs, and to remedy weakness of yang in the body.

Warmth prescriptions are divided into three main groups:

(a) Those which warm the meridians and dispel cold from them.

(b) Those which warm the internal organs and dispel cold from them.

(c) Those which restore yang and correct mischannelling or incorrect direction of energy in the meridians.

Internal-warmth prescriptions are used to restore mental energies, to correct faulty internal distribution of energy and to aid the circulation and the digestive system. In the main they have a stimulating effect upon the bodily functions which helps to improve their workings. They are used in the treatment of dyspepsia (indigestion), ulcers, chilblains, and rheumatoid arthritis. An example of prescriptions of this type is Chinese Angelica Zi Yi Tonic (21). Another is Five Combination Tonic (22), whose main purpose is to restore Ch'i and improve the circulation. Experienced medical practitioners, when confronted with a patient who complains of pains in the abdomen accompanied by coldness, a pale tongue and a slow, weak pulse, will usually prescribe Li Chung Pills (23) to restore central Ch'i. According to the individual case, other herbs may be added, such as aconitum or cinnamon. For those experiencing bowel problems, golden thread (*Coptis chinensis*) may be added. Each new combination has a separate name. In order to stop vomiting in patients suffering from the aforementioned symptoms, and in the treatment of ulcers, heart disease, high blood pressure and liver disease, Euodia Tonic (24) is used.

For some minor complaints, such as insect bites and rashes, single herbs are prescribed in the form of ointments and oils. Herbal medicine practitioners do not usually deal with injuries, except to prescribe medicine which clears blood clotting and bruises. This is also used for the treatment of broken bones; in addition, broken limbs are generally set with bamboo splints and a poultice of herbs applied.

THE PREPARATION OF PRESCRIPTIONS

The most common method of preparing Chinese herbal medicine is to make a soup or tea (t'ang). Alternatively the herbs are pulverized and rolled in a small quantity of a moistening agent such as honey to form pills, or are finely powdered and added to warm water.

The quantities given in each prescription are for one dose of medicine unless otherwise stated. In the case of soups, the ingredients are simmered in a non-metallic (usually clay) pot with a given quantity of water. When the liquid has reduced to a stated amount, the soup is ready to drink. Quantities of water are given in rice bowls, as this is the standard measure.

Where the herbs need to be ground, made into pills or stir-fried, this will be done by the herbalist. The only part of the preparation normally done at home is the boiling of herbs to make a soup.

NOTE ON THE NAMES OF HERBS

The common English (or in some cases, Chinese) name, where available, has generally been given for the herbs used in these prescriptions, with the botanical (Latin) equivalent in brackets. Many of the herbs used are not native to Britain and hence have no common English equivalent for the botanical name. For some very well-known herbs, the botanical name has been omitted.

INDIVIDUAL PRESCRIPTIONS

1 Ma Huang Soup

Symptoms High fever, stuffy or running nose, headache, general achiness, white tongue, floating pulse. This prescription is used to treat these symptoms when associated with coldness.

9 g ma huang (*Ephedra vulgaris*)
9 g cinnamon
9 g apricot kernels (*Prunus armeniaca*)
6 g liquorice (*Glycyrrhiza glabra*)

Preparation The liquorice is stir-fried in honey. Add it to the other ingredients in 3 rice bowls of water. Reduce the soup by simmering until ¾ rice bowl of liquid remains.

2 Cinnamon Soup

Symptoms High fever, stuffy or running nose, headache, aches all over the body, white tongue, floating pulse, all associated with coldness.

9 g cinnamon
9 g peony (*Paeonia lactiflora*)
2 slices ginger (*Zingiber officinale*)
4 Chinese jujubes (*Zizyphus jujuba*)
6 g liquorice (*Glycyrrhiza glabra*)

Preparation Add the ingredients to 3 rice bowls of water and reduce by simmering until ¾ rice bowl of liquid remains.

3 Honeysuckle and Forsythia Powder

Symptoms High fever, stuffy or running nose, headache, pain over the whole body, white tongue and floating pulse associated with heat.

9 g honeysuckle (*Lonicera japonica*)
9 g weeping forsythia (*Forsythia suspensa*)
6 g great burdock (*Arctium lappa*)
6 g balloon flower (*Platycodon grandiflorus*)
5 g mint (*Mentha arvensis*)
6 g soybean (*Glycine max*)
6 g liquorice (*Glycyrrhiza glabra*)
6 g tan chu (*Lophatherum gracile*)
6 g *Schizonepeta tenuifolia*

Preparation   The herbs are ground to a fine powder. You can add this to warm water and drink it, or it can be put into a capsule. These quantities provide three doses, which should be taken over the course of a day.

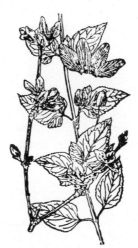

*Forsythia
suspensa*

4   Mulberry and Chrysanthemum Drink

Symptoms   High fever, stuffy or running nose, headache, pain over the whole body, white tongue and floating pulse associated with heat. This very pleasant-tasting preparation is a popular family medication usually used in summer and autumn.

9 g mulberry leaves (*Morus alba*)
6 g chrysanthemum (*Chrysanthemum indicum*)
6 g mint (*Mentha arvensis*)

18 g weeping forsythia (*Forsythia suspensa*)
9 g balloon flower (*Platycodon grandiflorus*)
9 g apricot kernels (*Prunus armeniaca*)
18 g common reed (*Phragmites communis*)
3 g liquorice (*Glycyrrhiza glabra*)

Preparation Add the ingredients to 3 rice bowls of water and reduce by simmering until ¾ rice bowl of liquid remains. This provides one dose. The herbs can be boiled a second time to provide another dose.

5   Cimicifuga and Pueraria Soup

Symptoms Used for children under the age of five and adults suffering from chickenpox or measles if the rash associated with the disease is slow to appear.

6 g *Cimicifuga dahurica*
15 g *Pueraria lobata*
9 g peony (*Paeonia lactiflora*)
9 g liquorice (*Glycyrrhiza glabra*)

Preparation Add the ingredients to 3 rice bowls of water and reduce by simmering until ¾ rice bowl of liquid remains. This provides one dose which should be taken each day for three days.

6   Ma Huang and Cinnamon Soup

Symptoms Swelling of the head, heaviness of the body, pain, white tongue, slow and floating pulse, moist appearance, all caused by cold-winded and wetness-related illnesses.

9 g ma huang (*Ephedra vulgaris*)
9 g cinnamon
9 g apricot kernels (*Prunus armeniaca*)
6 g liquorice (*Glycyrrhiza glabra*)
9 g *Atractylis chinensis*

Preparation The liquorice is first stir-fried in honey. Add the ingredients to 3 rice bowls of water and reduce by simmering until ¾ rice bowl of liquid remains. One dose should be taken each day after the evening meal.

7   Yer Pi Soup

Symptoms   Swollen body with wind and a floating pulse caused by yang water illnesses.

9 g ma huang (*Ephedra vulgaris*)
15 g gypsum
6 g liquorice (*Glycyrrhiza glabra*)
3 slices fresh ginger
3 Chinese jujubes (*Zizyphus jujuba*)

Preparation   Add the ingredients to 3 rice bowls of water and reduce by simmering until $\frac{3}{4}$ rice bowl of liquid remains. This provides one dose. Alternatively the herbs can be crushed to a powder with 6–9 g *Atractylis chinensis* to make Yer Pi Powder. The powder can be added to warm water or made into capsules, and provides two to three doses.

8   Prescription to Expel Wind and Promote the Passage of Water

Symptoms   Swollen body with wind and floating pulse in the elderly and women.

9 g *Spirodela polyrrhiza*
9 g *Perilla frutescens*
12 g mulberry root cortex (*Morus alba*)
30 g Siberian motherwort (*Leonurus sibiricus*)
12 g plantain (*Plantago paludosa*)
30 g *Imperata cylindrica*
18 g honeysuckle (*Lonicera caprifolium*)
18 g weeping forsythia (*Forsythia suspensa*)
6 g liquorice (*Glycyrrhiza glabra*)

Preparation   Add the ingredients to $4\frac{1}{2}$ rice bowls of water and reduce by simmering until 1 bowl of liquid remains.

9   Da Zhang Qi Soup

Symptoms   Hard stools, bloated and painful abdomen, high temperature, thirst, headache, delirium and vomiting of blood.

9 g medicinal rhubarb (*Rheum officinale*)
12 g sodium sulphate
9 g magnolia (*Magnolia officinalis*)
9 g Seville orange (*Citrus aurantium*)

Preparation   Add the ingredients to 3 rice bowls of water and reduce by simmering until 1 rice bowl of liquid remains.

10   Lian Gor Powder

Symptoms   Hard stools, bloated and painful abdomen, high temperature, thirst, headache, delirium and vomiting of blood.

6 g medicinal rhubarb (*Rheum officinale*)
9 g sodium sulphate
9 g skullcap (*Scutellaria baicalensis*)
9 g jasmine (*Jasminum paniculatum*)
18 g weeping forsythia (*Forsythia suspensa*)
6 g bamboo leaves (*Lopatherum gracile*)
6 g menthol
15 g honey
3 g liquorice (*Glycyrrhiza glabra*)

Preparation   The ingredients are ground to a powder. Add this to warm water, or it can be made into capsules. These quantities provide three to four doses, to be taken over the course of a day.

11   Warm Spleen Soup

Symptoms   Hardness of the bowels, coldness in the limbs and a sinking, slow pulse caused by coldness in the spleen. Expansion of the bowels and constipation caused by concentrated yin cold.

9 g *Aconitum balfourii* or *A. chinense*
6 g dried ginger
9 g *Campanumoea pilosula*
3 g liquorice (*Glycyrrhiza glabra*)
9 g medicinal rhubarb (*Rheum officinale*)

Preparation   Add the ingredients to 3 rice bowls of water and reduce by simmering until $\frac{3}{4}$ rice bowl of liquid remains.

12   Rhubarb and Aconitum Soup

Symptoms   Hardness of the bowels, coldness in the limbs and a sinking, slow pulse, or expansion of the bowels and constipation.

> 9 g medicinal rhubarb (*Rheum officinale*)
> 9 g *Aconitum balfourii* or *A. chinense*
> 6 g wild ginger (*Asarum sieboldii*)

Preparation   Add the ingredients to 3 rice bowls of water and reduce by simmering until ¾ rice bowl of liquid remains.

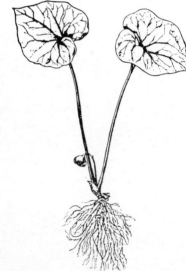

Asarum sieboldii

13   Wu Yan Pills

Symptoms   Dryness after illness or in old age. Weakness in the blood affecting the bowels after childbirth. Persistent hardness of bowel movements.

> 9 g *Prunus consociiflora*
> 9 g pine kernels (*Pinus armandii*)
> 9 g *Biota orientalis*
> 12 g apricot kernels (*Prunus armeniaca*)
> 9 g peach kernels (*Prunus persica*)
> 9 g tangerine peel (*Citrus reticulata*)

Preparation   The herbs are ground to a powder and mixed with honey to make a large pill. This pill should be chewed rather than swallowed whole. Alternatively, several smaller pills may be made.

14   Ten Jujubes Soup

Symptoms   Concentration of moisture in the chest or gathering of fluids in the body, swollen abdomen, yellow tongue.

   0·5 g *Euphorbia kansuensis*
   0·5 g *Euphorbia pekinensis*
   0·5 g *Daphne genkwa*
   10 Chinese jujube (*Zizyphus jujuba*)

Preparation   Remove the stones from the jujubs and crush them. Add all the ingredients to $4\frac{1}{2}$–5 rice bowls of water and simmer until 1–$1\frac{1}{2}$ rice bowls of liquid remain. A very swift-acting medicine.

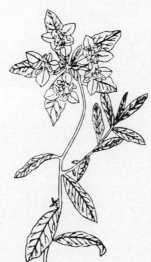

Euphorbia pekinensis

15   Bupleurum Tonic

Symptoms   Fluctuating heat and coldness, fullness in the chest, loss of appetite, bitter taste in the mouth, dry throat and dizziness. (This medicine is so popular that there is a Chinese poem about it.)

18 g *Bupleurum chinense*
12 g skullcap (*Scutellaria baicalensis*)
12 g *Campanumoea pilosula*
9 g *Pinellia ternata*
3 slices fresh ginger
3 Chinese jujubes (*Zizyphus jujuba*)
6 g liquorice (*Glycyrrhiza glabra*)

Preparation   Add the ingredients to 3 rice bowls of water and reduce by simmering until $\frac{3}{4}$ rice bowl of liquid remains.

16   Chao Yan Powder

Symptoms   Bloating of chest and waist, loss of appetite, bowel disorders, loss of spirit.

9 g *Bupleurum chinense*
9 g peony (*Paeonia lactiflora*)
9 g Chinese angelica (*Angelica sinensis*)
9 g *Atractylis macrocephala*
9 g Indian bread (*Poria cocos*)
6 g fresh ginger
6 g liquorice (*Glycyrrhiza glabra*)

Preparation   The liquorice is stir-fried in honey. All the herbs can then be ground into a powder, which can be taken in warm water or put into capsules. This gives a day's treatment of three doses. Alternatively add the ingredients to 3 rice bowls of water and reduce by simmering until $\frac{3}{4}$ rice bowl of liquid remains. This makes one dose, to be taken each day.

17   Zi Yi Tonic

Symptoms   As for Chao Yan Powder (16).

15 g *Aconitum balfourii* or *A. chinense*
12 g dried ginger
15 g liquorice (*Glycyrrhiza glabra*)

Preparation The liquorice is stir-fried in honey. Add all the ingredients to 3–3½ rice bowls of water and reduce by simmering until ¾ rice bowl of liquid remains.

18   Pain and Diarrhoea Prescription

Symptoms As Chao Yan Powder (16).

12 g *Atractylis macrocephala*
12 g peony (*Paeonia lactiflora*)
9 g tangerine peel (*Citrus reticulata*)
6 g *Stenocoelium divaricatum* root

Preparation Add the ingredients to 3 rice bowls of water and reduce by simmering until ¾ rice bowl of liquid remains.

19   Huang Lian Soup

Symptoms Concentration of heat, feeling of nausea without actual vomiting, abdominal pain. Diarrhoea accompanied by dizziness and weakness.

6 g golden thread (*Coptis chinensis*)
9 g *Pinellia ternata*
6 g dried ginger
6 g cinnamon
15 g *Campanumoea pilosula*
4 Chinese jujubes (*Zizyphus jujuba*)
15 g liquorice (*Glycyrrhiza glabra*)

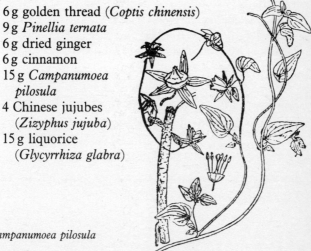

Campanumoea pilosula

Preparation The liquorice is stir-fried in honey. Add the ingredients to 3 rice bowls of water and reduce by simmering until ¾ rice bowl of liquid remains.

20   Seven Wonder Tonic

Symptoms   Used for malaria. Fluctuations of heat and cold, fullness at chest and waist, nausea.

- 3 g basak (*Dichroa febrifuga*)
- 3 g magnolia (*Magnolia officinalis*)
- 3 g green tangerine peel (*Citrus reticulata*)
- 3 g tangerine peel (*Citrus reticulata*)
- 3 g liquorice (*Glycyrrhiza glabra*)
- 9 g betel nut (*Areca catechu*)
- 3 g *Amomum tsaoko*

Preparation   Add the ingredients to 3 rice bowls of water and reduce by simmering until $\frac{3}{4}$ rice bowl of liquid remains.

21   Chinese Angelica Zi Yi Tonic

Symptoms   Indigestion, pain from stomach ulcers, chilblains or rheumatoid arthritis.

- 9 g Chinese angelica (*Angelica sinensis*)
- 9 g cinnamon
- 9 g peony (*Paeonia lactiflora*)
- 3 g wild ginger (*Asarum sieboldii*)
- 6 g liquorice (*Glycyrrhiza glabra*)
- 9 g Chinese jujubes (*Zizyphus jujuba*)
- 6 g *Clematis armandii*

Preparation   Add the ingredients to $4\frac{1}{2}$ rice bowls of water and reduce by simmering until 1 rice bowl of liquid remains.

22   Five Combination Tonic

Symptoms   Indigestion, pain from stomach ulcers, chilblains, rheumatoid arthritis, poor circulation.

- 9 g milk vetch (*Astragalus membranaceus*)
- 9 g cinnamon
- 9 g peony (*Paeonia lactiflora*)
- 18 g fresh ginger

Preparation   Add the ingredients to $2\frac{1}{2}$ rice bowls of water and reduce by simmering until $\frac{3}{4}$ rice bowl of liquid remains.

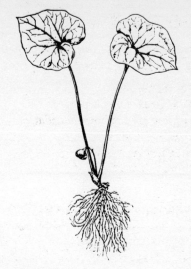

Asarum sieboldii

23 Li Chung Pill

Symptoms Coldness, pains in the abdomen, pale tongue and a slow, weak pulse.

   9 g dried ginger
   12 g *Atractylis chinensis*
   15 g *Campanumoea pilosula*
   6 g liquorice (*Glycyrrhiza glabra*)

Preparation The ingredients are ground into a powder and made into a large pill with honey. This pill should be chewed. Alternatively several smaller pills may be made.

24 Evodia Tonic

Symptoms Stomach ulcer. Prevention of vomiting in those suffering from bowel problems and abdominal pain.

   6 g *Evodia rutaecarpa*
   9 g fresh ginger
   15 g *Campanumoea pilosula*
   12 Chinese jujubes (*Zizyphus jujuba*)

Preparation Add the ingredients to 3 rice bowls of water and reduce by simmering until $\frac{3}{4}$ rice bowl of liquid remains.

25   San Hou Soup

Symptoms   Stuffy lung passages, cough, slight shortness of breath (but not asthma), coughing due to flu, whooping cough.

  6 g ma huang (*Ephedra sinica*)
  9 g apricot kernels (*Prunus armeniaca*)
  3 g liquorice (*Glycyrrhiza glabra*)

Preparation   Add the ingredients to 3 rice bowls of water and reduce by simmering until ¾ rice bowl of liquid remains.

26   Variation of Cinnamon Soup

Symptoms   Arthritic pain and swelling.

  9 g cinnamon
  9 g *Aconitum balfourii* or *A. chinense*
  6 g liquorice (*Glycyrrhiza glabra*)
  9 g fresh ginger
  3 Chinese jujubes (*Zizyphus jujuba*)

Preparation   Add the ingredients to 3 rice bowls of water and reduce by simmering until ¾ rice bowl of liquid remains.

27   Ling Kwei Zhu Chin Soup

Symptoms   Simple coughs in their early stages.

  18 g Indian bread (*Poria cocos*)
  9 g cinnamon
  12 g *Atractylis chinensis*
  9 g liquorice (*Glycyrrhiza glabra*)

Preparation   Add the ingredients to 3 rice bowls of water and reduce by simmering until ¾ rice bowl of liquid remains.

28   Eight Precious Soup

Symptoms   Pale face, dizziness, impaired vision, depression, reluctance to speak, loss of appetite, tongue pale with yellowish furring, pulse weak and difficult to find. Given to women as a tonic after childbirth and in the case of frayed nerves caused by stress.

15 g *Campanumoea pilosula*
12 g *Atractylis chinensis*
9 g Indian bread (*Poria cocos*)
6 g liquorice (*Glycyrrhiza glabra*)
12 g *Rehmannia glutinosa*
9 g Chinese angelica (*Angelica sinensis*)
12 g peony (*Paeonia lactiflora*)
6 g *Ligusticum acutilobum*

Preparation Add the ingredients to 6 rice bowls of water and reduce by simmering until 1½ rice bowls of liquid remaining.

Note: This prescription is a combination of Four Natural Products Tonic (29) and Four Gentlemen's Tonic (30).

29 Four Natural Products Tonic

Symptoms Menstrual disorder. Excessive kicking of foetus. Threatened miscarriage. Anaemia. Poor circulation. Loss of tone in the muscles of the womb, especially after childbirth. Blood-related symptoms, 'emptiness' of blood.

12 g *Rehmannia glutinosa*
9 g Chinese angelica (*Angelica sinensis*)
12 g peony (*Paeonia lactiflora*)
6 g *Ligusticum acutilobum*

Preparation Add the ingredients to 3 rice bowls of water and reduce by simmering until ¾ rice bowl of liquid remains.

30 Four Gentlemen's Tonic

Symptoms Weakness for no apparent reason, especially in very good weather. This prescription restores Ch'i in the blood.

15 g *Campanumoea pilosula*
12 g *Atractylis chinensis*
9 g Indian bread (*Poria cocos*)
6 g liquorice (*Glycyrrhiza glabra*)

Preparation Add the ingredients to 3 rice bowls of water and reduce by simmering until ¾ rice bowl of liquid remains.

31   Angelica and Peony Soup

Symptoms   Discomfort during pregnancy. Bruises and blood clots. Continuing pain in the abdomen which does not respond to other herbal remedies. Hardening of the arteries. Kidney problems in men. Depression. This prescription lowers cholesterol, restores the blood and treats the liver.

3 g Chinese angelica (*Angelica sinensis*)
5 g peony (*Paeonia lactiflora*)
2 g *Ligusticum acutilobum*
3 g *Atractylis macrocephala*
3 g Indian bread (*Poria cocos*)
5 g water plantain (*Alisma plantago-aquatica*)

Preparation   Add the ingredients to 3 rice bowls of water and reduce by simmering until ¾ rice bowl of liquid remains. Alternatively the ingredients can be crushed to a powder and taken as three doses with warm water or in capsules.

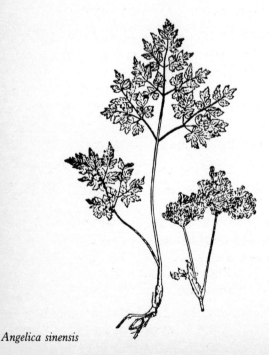

Angelica sinensis

32   Peony and Liquorice Soup

Symptoms   Kidney pains. Tiredness and exhaustion in women. Pains in the hips in women.

10 g peony (*Paeonia lactiflora*)
10 g liquorice (*Glycyrrhiza glabra*)
2 g *Corydalis turtschaninovii*

Preparation   Add the ingredients to 3 rice bowls of water and reduce by simmering until ¾ rice bowl of liquid remains. This makes two doses.

33   Increase of Dew Soup

Symptoms   Constipation. High fever, extreme thirst, tongue very dry and red, very hard stools, slow pulse. These symptoms usually occur in summer. This very powerful medicine is used mainly for yang and hot diseases, and provides dew, dispels hotness and moistens the intestines.

10 g figwort (*Scrophularia nodosa*)
8 g *Ophiopogon japonica*
8 g *Rehmannia glutinosa*

Preparation   Add the ingredients to 3 rice bowls of water and reduce by simmering until ¾ rice bowl of liquid remains.

34   Cinnamon and Peony Soup

Symptoms   Chilblains. This soup is curative and preventative, keeping the body warm. It should be taken for five consecutive days, or ten if the chilblains start to burst.

3 g cinnamon
3 g peony (*Paeonia lactiflora*)
2 g Chinese angelica (*Angelica sinensis*)
4 Chinese jujubes (*Zizyphus jujuba*)
2 g liquorice (*Glycyrrhiza glabra*)

Preparation   The liquorice is stir-fried in honey. Add the ingredients to 3 rice bowls of water and reduce by simmering until ¾ rice bowl of liquid remains.

35 San Sheng Yin

Symptoms Excess of sputum. This prescription is also commonly prescribed in the treatment of paralysis. Recently it has been used to relieve unbearable pain such as that caused by cancer. It has a powerful painkilling effect, but for this purpose should be boiled for a much longer time in order to limit the powerfulness of the three main herbs.

4 g *Arisaema thunbergii*
4 g *Aconitum balfourii* or *A. chinense* main root
3 g *Aconitum fischeri*
3 g costus (*Saussurea lappa*)
24 g ginger
9 g ginseng

Preparation Boil all the ingredients except the costus in 3–4 rice bowls of water for 1–2 hours. The liquid should reduce to 1 rice bowl in quantity. Add the costus a few minutes before the end of boiling.

36 Zhi Sou San

Symptoms Irritating cough at night. Cough caused by flu. This prescription expands the lungs and dispels phlegm.

4 g *Schizonepeta tenuifolia*
3 g peeled tangerine skin (*Citrus reticulata*)
9 g *Stemona japonica* or *S. sessilifolia* or *S. tuberosa*
9 g bai gian (*Cynanchum stauntoni*)
9 g *Aster amellus*
9 g balloon flower (*Platycodon grandiflorus*)
3 g liquorice (*Glycyrrhiza glabra*)

Preparation The herbs are ground into a powder and added to water to be drunk. Alternatively boil them whole with 3–4 rice bowls of water until the liquid has reduced to ¾ bowl in quantity, to be taken while warm.

37 Three Seeds Cough-Smothering Soup

Symptoms Coughs, difficulty in breathing, phlegm, stuffy chest. Restores the incorrect flow of Ch'i in the channels;

mainly used for the elderly. Used in the treatment of bronchitis.

9 g *Perilla frutescens* seeds
9 g mustard seeds
9 g radish seeds

Preparation   Add the ingredients to 3 rice bowls of water and reduce by simmering until ¾ rice bowl of liquid remains.

38   Jian Chi Soup

Symptoms   Cold cough, cold phlegm. Cough which causes difficulty in breathing at night.

9 g *Perilla frutescens* seeds
9 g *Pinellia ternata*
6 g *Angelica decursiva*
6 g magnolia (*Magnolia officinalis*)
3 g dried tangerine peel (*Citrus reticulata*)
9 g Chinese angelica (*Angelica sinensis*)
1·5 g cinnamon
9 g sliced fresh ginger
3 g liquorice (*Glycyrrhiza glabra*)

Preparation   Boil all ingredients except the cinnamon in 3 rice bowls of water until ¾ bowl of liquid remains. Crush the cinnamon into a powder and place in a bowl. Pour the boiled medicine over the cinnamon.

39   Soup to Mend Yang and Restore the Elements

Symptoms   Partial paralysis after a stroke, with facial distortion, lack of control over speech, saliva, bowels and bladder. The last five ingredients help to move the blood and to dispel blood clots. Dried earthworm is sometimes added to this prescription. It is believed to help the blood move, in the same way that a worm moves through the earth.

30–60 g milk vetch (*Astragalus membranaceus*)
6 g Chinese angelica (*Angelica sinensis*)
9 g peony (*Paeonia lactiflora*) (unpeeled)
6 g *Ligustrum wallichii*
9 g peach kernel (*Prunus persica*)
4·5 g safflower

Preparation Add the ingredients to 5–6 rice bowls of water and reduce by simmering until 1½ rice bowls of liquid remain.

40   Ginger and White Carrot

Symptoms Chronic bronchitis accompanied by tightness in the chest and dry stools. This prescription will relieve much of the discomfort, although it may not effect a complete cure.

15 g fresh ginger
6 slices white carrot
30 g honey

Preparation Add the ingredients to 3 rice bowls of water and reduce by simmering until ¾ rice bowl of liquid remains. Take the whole mixture once per day for five to seven days.

41   Apricot Kernel and White Carrot Powder

Symptoms Coughs and tightness in the chest and shortness of breath, when it is difficult to get rid of phlegm. This prescription is not effective for persistent coughs, but it is easily made and will often cure a mild cough which is at an early stage.

10 apricot kernels (*Prunus armeniaca*)
10 slices white carrot

Preparation The two ingredients are crushed together to a powder and divided into two equal portions to be taken during the course of a day. The powder is taken orally in red-sugared water.

42   Anemarrhena and Coltsfoot

Symptoms Coughs in the elderly accompanied by an excess of phlegm, shortness of breath and slight asthmatic symptoms.

Coltsfoot is well known as a cough remedy. Culpeper says of it: 'Called also Cough-wort ... The fresh leaves, or juice, or syrup thereof, is good for a hot, dry cough, or wheezing, and shortness of breath. The dry leaves are best for those who have thin rheums and distillations upon their lungs, causing a cough; for which also ... the root is very good.'[22]

10 g *Anemarrhena asphodeloides*
10 g coltsfoot (*Tussilago farfara*)
6 g imperial fritillary (*Fritillaria verticillata*)
5 Chinese jujubes (*Zizyphus jujuba*)
3 slices fresh ginger

Preparation   The first two ingredients are stir-fried in honey. Add the ingredients to 3 rice bowls of water and reduce by simmering until ¾ rice bowl of liquid remains. This makes two doses, which is one day's treatment. Alternatively the ingredients are crushed to a powder, in which case 6 g should be taken twice a day in water or as capsules.

43   Plum and Sweet Pear

Symptoms   Chronic bronchitis with shortness of breath and rapid breathing, with persistent phlegm.

3 plums
1 sweet pear

Preparation   Roast the plums over a flame until the outer layer is burned; then peel off the skin and discard it. Crush the fruit and place in the pear which has been sliced open; this is steamed and eaten. One should be taken per night.

44   Cold Remedy

Symptoms   Colds with high fever, headache and aching of the whole body. (This is a very ancient prescription which has been handed down by word of mouth.)

9 g *Perilla acuta*
9 g *Stenocoelium divaricatum*
9 g *Schizonepeta tenuifolia*
6 g peppermint (*Mentha piperita*)

Preparation   Add the ingredients to 3 rice bowls of water and reduce by simmering until ¾ rice bowl of liquid remains. In winter and spring, add red sugar and fresh ginger. In summer and autumn, add bamboo leaves and white sugar.

45   Ma Huang and Apricot Kernel Soup

Symptoms   Influenza in winter and spring, with a high temperature, cough, shortness of breath and phlegm. Depresses coughs and dispels phlegm.

> 6 g ma huang (*Ephedra vulgaris*)
> 10 g apricot kernels (*Prunus armeniaca*)
> 3 g red tea
> 6 g *Perilla frutescens*
> 3 g liquorice (*Glycyrrhiza glabra*)
> 3 slices fresh ginger

Preparation   Add the ingredients to 3 rice bowls of water and reduce by simmering until ¾ rice bowl of liquid remains. Take after a meal.

46   Plantain and Honeysuckle Soup

Symptoms   Summer and autumn diarrhoea. Culpeper says that plantain 'stays all manner of fluxes.'[22]

> 30 g plantain (*Plantago sibirica, P. depressa*)
> 30 g honeysuckle (*Lonicera japonica*)

Preparation   Add the ingredients with red and white sugar to 3 rice bowls of water and reduce by simmering until ¾ rice bowl of liquid remains. This makes two doses, to be taken during the course of a day.

47   Roast Garlic

Symptoms   Diarrhoea with abdominal pains which has persisted for three to five days.

> 1 large bulb garlic

Preparation   Roast in a flame. Take one freshly roasted bulb per day.

48   Ginger and Spring Onion Soup

Symptoms   Colds with headache, high temperature, cough, phlegm and a running nose, especially in winter. This prescription is a popular home remedy.

10 g fresh ginger
1 large fresh spring onion, whole
3 g Japanese prickly ash (*Zanthoxylum piperitum*)
30 g outer skin of white carrot

Preparation   Boil the ingredients for 20–30 minutes in 1 small rice bowl of water. The brew is taken while still hot to promote light sweating.

49   Chrysanthemum and Peppermint

Symptoms   Red and painful eyes which are watering and causing impaired vision.

10 g wild chrysanthemum
3 g peppermint (*Menta piperita*)
6 g *Tribulus terrestris*

Preparation   The herbs used should be fresh if possible. Add the ingredients to 3 rice bowls of water and reduce by simmering until $\frac{3}{4}$ rice bowl of liquid remains. Take by mouth; the liquid is also used warm to bathe the eyes.

50   Stenocoelium and Schizonepeta Soup

Symptoms   Intermittent toothache.

6 g *Stenocoelium divaricatum*
6 g *Schizonepeta tenuifolia*
6 g chrysanthemum
6 g balloon flower (*Platycodon grandiflorus*)
6 g *Ligustrum wallichii*
6 g *Aconitum balfourii* or *A. chinense*
6 g *Aconitum kusnezoffii*
10 g figwort (*Scrophularia nodosa*)
3 g liquorice (*Glycyrrhiza glabra*)

Preparation   Add the ingredients to 3 rice bowls of water and reduce by simmering until ¾ rice bowl of liquid remains. Take for three days.

51   Pregnancy Test

Symptoms   This prescription is used as a test for pregnancy when a period is overdue and no accompanying discomfort is felt. If the patient is pregnant, the prescription will have no ill effects; if she is not, it will cause the period to start.

9 g *Ligustrum wallichii*
9 g *Angelica dahurica*
6 g *Schizonepeta tenuifolia*
10 g *Atractylis macrocephala*
6 g skullcap (*Scutellaria baicalensis*)
6 g *Perilla frutescens*
10 g Chinese angelica (*Angelica sinensis*)
6 g liquorice (*Glycyrrhiza glabra*)

Preparation   Add the ingredients to 3 rice bowls of water and reduce by simmering until ¾ rice bowl of liquid remains. Reboil the herbs three times a day.

52   Rubia and Red Sugar

Symptoms   This prescription is used for women who are not pregnant and whose period is two to three months overdue, accompanied by pain, with fever and coldness. The prescription should not be continued once the period starts.

30 g *Rubia cordifolia* root
30 g red sugar

Preparation   Add the rubia to 3 rice bowls of water and reduce by simmering until ¾ rice bowl of liquid remains. Add the sugar. Take while still warm once a day for three to five days.

53   Ginseng and Aconitum Soup

Symptoms   Cold hands and feet, cold, heavy sweating with tasteless sweat, very weak pulse. This very expensive prescription helps to restore yang, giving strength to the heart and raising the blood pressure. It is used especially for those over the age of fifty with a tendency to faint and helps to cope with hardening of the arteries.

12 g ginseng
9 g *Aconitum balfourii* or *A. chinense*

Preparation   Add the ingredients to 3 rice bowls of water and reduce by simmering until ¾ rice bowl of liquid remains.

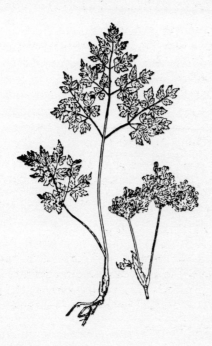

Angelica sinensis

6

MEDICINAL FOODS

In the early day of Chinese medicine there was a branch known as 'medicinal diet' or, literally, 'eat medicine'. This branch is believed to have been responsible for the idea that certain foods should be eaten at different times of the year.

The influence of this branch of medicine persists to the present day. The Chinese are very fond of medicinal soups, suitable for the whole family, which are taken as special treats. Different types of soup are made according to the time of year.

It is impossible to give precise recipes as quantities and, to some extent, ingredients vary from family to family. Generally, quantities of soup are gauged according to the number of people who will be eating, while the quantities of the herbal ingredients remain fairly constant. Cooking time is generally judged by the time necessary to cook the main food ingredient.

Lotus Seed, Lily and Lean Pork Soup

Lotus seeds are useful for strengthening the spleen and stomach; they promote mental stability and healthy functioning of the kidneys. They are used to treat males suffering from wet dreams and seminal emission, females with excessive menstrual loss and leucorrhoea and those suffering from diarrhoea.

Lily is used to treat dry lungs and dry coughs, to restore central Ch'i, to strengthen the kidneys, to treat problems of heart, lungs, spleen and stomach, to dispel hotness and stop coughs, and as a valuable tonic in the treatment of tuberculosis. It is also used to treat neurasthenia.

The combination of lotus seeds and lily contains large amounts of vitamin C and protein and is very popular.

Lotus Seed and Lily Soup, a sweet soup, is presented at the

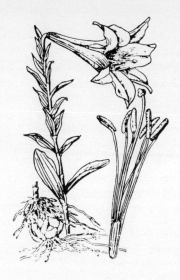

Lilium
brownii

end of wedding banquets, because the names in Chinese form a pun on 'continuous sons' and 'a hundred together', hence wishing the couple a hundred years of married life with many sons.

Preparation   Make a soup with lean pork to which are added:

15–24 g lotus seeds
15–30 g lily (*Lilium brownii*)

Chinese Yam and Chinese Wolfberry Soup

Yam has the ability to strengthen the spleen and stomach, and the lungs and kidneys, and contains large quantities of protein and carbohydrate.

Wolfberry seeds aid in the restoration of the liver and kidneys and are used in the treatment of diabetes.

Preparation   Make a meat soup with whatever lean meat is preferred, to which are added:

18–30 g Chinese yam (*Dioscorea batatas*)
6–15 g Chinese wolfberry seeds (*Lycium chinense*)

Boiled Eggs with *Loranthus parasiticus*

Loranthus parasiticus is used to treat liver and kidney complaints, to strengthen tendon muscles, in the preservation of blood, to dispel wind, to prevent threatened miscarriage and to promote the flow of breast milk. It is often employed in the treatment of rheumatism, back pain and loss of sensation in the limbs; it is also recommended for use in diabetes and high blood pressure caused by arteriosclerosis.

According to the classics of Chinese medicine, it is very helpful in relieving back pain in pregnant women. Many people use the herb on its own as a tea to prevent illness.

It also nourishes skin, muscles and hair and strengthens the teeth.

Preparation   Hard boil eggs in water containing 15–30 g *Loranthus parasiticus*. Eat the eggs and drink the water in which they were boiled.

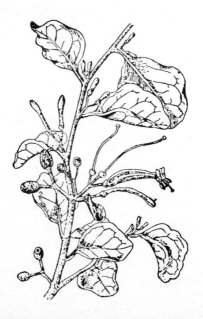

Loranthus parasiticus

Chinese Angelica and Lamb

Chinese angelica (*Angelica sinensis*) is regarded as the foremost herb for the treatment of gynaecological problems. As long as 2000 years ago, the medical treatise *Shen-nung Pen Ts'ao Chingar* [24] acclaimed its efficacy in treating female complaints, especially those related to menstruation.

Lamb, as well as its use in flavouring a dish, has its own medicinal qualities. It is said to give warmth to the spleen and stomach, to restore Ch'i and blood, providing health and strength to the body.

A prescription for angelica, ginger and lamb is given by the famous doctor Chang Chung Ching in his medical book;[25] it is said to relieve the pain experienced by women after childbirth.

9–15 g Chinese angelica (*Angelica sinensis*)
1 lb lamb
ginger slices to taste

Preparation Steam all the ingredients together in a cook pot (see p. 51) until the lamb is tender.

Pig's Kidneys and Tu Chung

There is a popular Chinese verse: 'Pain at waist – pig's kidney and tu chung.' It refers to the idea of using the corresponding organ of an animal to treat an organ in the human body.

Amongst its many uses tu chung protects the liver and kidneys, strengthens tendons and bones, and is a remedy for back pain. It is very effective in lowering blood pressure and cholesterol levels and is frequently used for these purposes. It is better taken fried than raw, but is best boiled. It is helpful in preventing threatened miscarriage in the middle stages of pregnancy.

1 pig's kidney
9–15 g tu chung bark (*Eucommia ulmoides*)

Preparation Steam together in a cook pot (see p. 51) until the kidney is cooked.

Ligustrum wallichii and Honey Stew

Coughing through the door, Doctor's eyebrows become creased.

This saying points up the fact that a cough can be the result of a variety of different causes. When a cough has persisted for some time and other medicine has not worked, this recipe is used.

6–12 g *Ligustrum wallichii* (3–6 g if powdered)
15–30 g honey

Preparation   Steam in a cook pot (see p. 51) for one hour.

Juice of Chinese Chives and Ginger with Milk

Chives taste hot and provide warmth; they are associated with the liver, stomach and kidney meridians and activate Ch'i.

Ginger also tastes hot and provides warmth; it is associated with the lung, stomach and spleen meridians. It dispels cold, stops vomiting and disperses sputum.

Milk has a sweet taste and is associated with the lung and stomach meridians. This recipe is used to treat an upset stomach and vomiting immediately after eating.

2 soup-spoons juice from fresh chives
1 teaspoon juice from fresh ginger
250 ml fresh milk

Preparation   Steam together in a cook pot (see p. 51) and take before a meal.

Watercress and Date Soup

This recipe is used to treat a dry cough, dry throat and constipation. Watercress, as well as containing an abundance of vitamins A, C and D, has the ability to clear and moisten the lungs. Dates are sweet and provide dew.

500 g watercress
5–6 dates

Preparation   Add water and boil for a lengthy period, up to two hours or even longer.

Chicken with *Polygonum multiflorum*

This dish nourishes the blood and strengthens the kidneys. It is popularly used to treat problems of the uterus and haemorrhoids. As well as its other effects, it keeps the hair black and shiny.

30 g *Polygonum multiflorum*
one 500 g chicken

Preparation Extract the internal organs from the chicken. Grind the herb to a powder and wrap it in several layers of white muslin. Put this inside the chicken, add water and boil until the meat falls away from the bones. Remove the packet of powder. Add salt, oil, ginger and wine to taste. Drink the soup and eat the chicken.

ACUPUNCTURE AND
MOXIBUSTION

Westerners are becoming (in theory at least) quite well acquainted with Chinese acupuncture. Or, rather, they think they are. For this area above all other areas of Chinese medicine has been misunderstood and misused by Westerners. Readers may wonder why a herbal book has a chapter on acupuncture and moxibustion. Quite simply, it is usual in China to use all three methods together to relieve symptoms. That this is little known in the West is a major reason for the patchy success of acupuncture outside China.

The term for acupuncture is Chen Chiu. This means literally 'needle moxi' – needle and heat. Acupuncture, using slim needles to reach the meridian lines, can be very effective by itself. However, heat will usually be used as well. This provides greater stimulation than the needles alone and is done by burning cone-shaped pieces of moxa wool (a soft, fluffy material made from the leaves of *Artemisia vulgaris*) on or near the skin or by applying heat from cigar-shaped sticks of the wool. Both methods complement, or in chronic cases supplant, acupuncture in affecting the flow of Ch'i and blood as influenced by the meridians. (This method is not commonly used by Westerners; perhaps the rather powerful smell of moxa puts them off.)

The same is true with regard to herbal prescriptions. Acupuncture and moxibustion play with powerful forces in the body. The body is less affected by this than, say, by a general anaesthetic using gas or drugs. However, it is nevertheless disturbed. Therefore herbal prescriptions, appropriate to the particular meridian or area of the body being treated, are recommended by all major books on this subject; in many cases herbalists will also be trained acupuncture/moxibustion-ists, and vice versa.

DIABETES

It is estimated that there are 50,000,000 sufferers from diabetes in the world today. The incidence of diabetes in Europe is between 20 and 40 per 1000 people, while in America it is as high as 50 per 1000.

This illness, which can be dangerous or even fatal if not properly controlled, was known to the Chinese as long ago as the T'ang dynasty, when it was observed that the urine of diabetics attracts ants (this sweetness of the urine is reflected in the Latin term for the complaint, diabetes mellitus, or sugar diabetes). Most diabetics are sufferers from the comparatively mild form of diabetes which usually occurs in middle age (maturity-onset diabetes). They are often overweight. The Chinese describe the symptoms as the three evaporations: the patient eats more, drinks more and urinates more. He also feels rather weak.

Mild cases of diabetes can be treated by diet without medicine. One method used by the Chinese is known as the 'boiled three times vegetables' diet. This gives a great deal of bulk and thus makes the patient feel full, without eating large amounts of protein. Any vegetables may be used, and these are chopped up and boiled in water for fifteen minutes. The water is poured away, fresh water is added and the vegetables are again boiled for fifteen minutes. This is repeated once more. The water is then squeezed from the vegetables before they are eaten.

As well as using this method, the eating of tomatoes, pumpkins, white cabbage and celery is highly recommended. Bitter melon is another recommended vegetable, and one which is very popular in China, especially in the south. Between 300 and 600 g of bitter melon should be taken at each meal in place of other vegetables. Onion is also recommended, in amounts of 50–100 g twice daily, boiled in water for no more than two minutes.

The Chinese also recognize the importance of exercise in reducing blood sugar: unlike medicine, exercise lowers the blood sugar level without side effects, and is particularly good for the slightly overweight middle-aged or elderly diabetic. Suggested sports are Chi Kung or Tai Chi, swimming, table tennis, badminton, volleyball, basketball and football. Exercise should be taken for twenty to thirty minutes every other day.

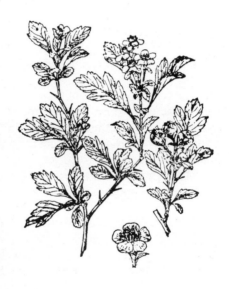

NOTES

1. Carmen Blacker, *The Catalpa Bow: A Study of Shamanistic Practices in Japan*, Cambridge University Press, 1975, chs. 12 and 15.
2. *Huang-ti Nei Ching Su Wen* (*The Yellow Emperor's Classic of Internal Medicine*), trans. Ilza Veith, University of Calfornia Press, 1949, 1972.
3. The Five Classics are the *I Ching* (*The Book of Changes*), the *Shu Ching* (*The Book of Historical Documents*), the *Shih Ching* (*The Book of Odes or Poetry*), the *Li Chi* (*The Record of Rites*) and the *Ch'un Ch'iu* (*Records or Annals of Spring and Autumn*).
4. See Ssu-ma Ch'ien, *Selection from the Records of the Historian*, trans. Yang Hsien-yi and Gladys Yang, Peking, 1979.
5. *Shoo King* (*The Book of Historical Documents*), trans. James Legge, in *The Chinese Classics*, Oxford University Press, 1871, vol. III; reprinted by Souther Materials Center Inc., Taipai, 1983.
6. *Shu Ching*, 'Charge to Yue', Part IV, Book 8, verse 1.8.
7. *Mencius*, trans. D. C. Lau, Penguin Books, 1940, Book III, Part A, p. 95.
8. Tso Ch'iu Ming, *Kuo Yu* (*The Discourse on the States*), *c.* 770–476 BCE. This work has not been completely translated into English, but the Chinese edition is available in the Needham Research Institute, Cambridge.
9. *Tso Chuan*, 'Duke Ch'eng – 10th Year'. The translation is based on the Chinese text in James Legge's *The Chinese Classics*, Oxford University Press, 1871, vol. V, p. 375; reprinted by Southern Materials Center Inc., Taipai, 1983.
10. Henri Doré, *Researches into Chinese Superstitions*, 15 vols., Walsh, 1914.
11. *Huang-ti Nei Ching Su Wen*, pp. 150–52.
12. Pan Ku *et al.*, *Chi'ien Han Shu*, *c.* 100 CE; Fan Yeh, *Hou Han Shou*, *c.* 450 CE. There is no complete English edition; Chinese editions are available in the Needham Research Institute, Cambridge.
13. Chang Chung Ching, *Shang Han Lun* (*Treatise on Febrile Diseases*), *c.* 200 CE. No full English translation exists; however, the Chinese edition is available in the Needham Research Institute, Cambridge.
14. Lao Tzu, *Tao Te Ching*: see D. C. Lau, *Lao Tzu*, Penguin Books, 1963; James Legge, *The Sacred Books of the East*, Oxford University Press, 1889, vol. XXXIX.
15. Shen-nung, *Shen-nung Pen Ts'ao Ching*, *c.* first century BCE.
16. *The Ramayana*, retold by William Buck, Mentor, 1978.

17. Kenneth Ch'en, *Buddhism in China*, Princeton University Press, 1972, p. 483.
18. Ch'en, op. cit., pp. 482–3.
19. Martin Palmer, *T'ung Shu: The Ancient Chinese Almanac*, Rider, 1986.
20. Li Shih-chen, *Pen Ts'ao Kang Mu* (*The Great Pharmacopoeia*), 1596 (posthumously published). The Chinese edition is available in the Needham Research Institute, Cambridge.
21. Peter Worsley, *Inside China*, Allen Lane, 1975.
22. Nicholas Culpeper, *The English Physitian*, 1652; published as *Culpeper's Complete Herbal*, W. Foulsham & Co., n.d., p. 97.
23. ibid., p. 274.
24. See note 15.
25. See note 13.

INDEX OF SYMPTOMS

migraine, 57
miscarriage, threatened, 57, 85
moistness, 75

nausea, 81, 82
 see also vomiting
nose, running, 59, 73, 74–5, 90
 stuffy, 73, 74–5

pain, 57, 61, 75, 82
paleness, 84–5
paralysis, *see* limbs
phlegm, 54, 88, 89, 90, 91, 92, 93
pregnancy, anaemia in, 85
 discomfort in, 86
 excessive kicking in, 85
 loss of muscular tone in, 85
 test for, 94
 threatened miscarriage, 57, 85
pulse, floating, 73, 74, 75, 76
 sinking, 77, 78
 slow, 75, 77, 78, 83
 weak, 83, 84–5, 94–5

skin complaints, 54, 61
spasms, 64
stomach ulcers, 82, 83
stools, dry, 90
stress, 84–5

sweating, 57, 59, 62, 94–5
swelling, 59, 61, 64, 75, 76

taste, bitter, 79–80
temperature, fluctuating, 79–80, 82
 high, 61, 73, 74–5, 76, 77, 87, 92,
 93
thirst, 61, 76, 77
throat, dry, 60, 79–80
 sore, 58, 62
tics, 64
tinnitus, 54, 58, 61
tiredness, 62, 87
tongue, dry, 87
 pale, 83, 84–5
 red, 61, 87
 yellow, 79, 84–5
toothache, 93–4

ulcers, stomach, 82, 83

vision, impaired, 57, 58, 84–5, 93
vomiting, 56, 61, 83
 see also nausea

waist, bloated, 80, 81, 82
weakness, 59, 81, 85
whooping cough, 55, 64, 84
wind, 76

Index of Herbs